Training Manual for Sight Without Eyes Through Mind and Perception

By Lloyd Hopkins

Training Manual for Sight Without Eyes Through Mind and Perception

By Lloyd Hopkins

Copyright 2008 by Clear Springs Press, LLC

Originally published in 1988

All rights reserved. Any copying or reprinting of this content requires the permission of the publisher.

ISBN-13: 978-1-884979-01-9
ISBN-10: 1-884979-01-7

BISAC Subject Headings:

OCC029000	**BODY, MIND & SPIRIT** / Unexplained Phenomena
OCC036000	**BODY, MIND & SPIRIT** / Spirituality / General
OCC019000	**BODY, MIND & SPIRIT** / Inspiration & Personal Growth
OCC000000	**BODY, MIND & SPIRIT** / General
SEL032000	**SELF-HELP** / Spiritual
SEL031000	**SELF-HELP** / Personal Growth / General
SEL000000	**SELF-HELP** / General
HEA037000	**HEALTH & FITNESS** / Vision

Any communications should be addressed to:

Clear Springs Press, LLC

http://www.clspress.com/contact.html

Table of Contents

Background		4
Dedication		8
Foreword		9
Introduction		11
Preface		15
Chapter 1	A Demonstration	16
Chapter 2	Mind Sight. What is it?	21
Chapter 3	A Research in Human Behavior	26
Chapter 4	The Beginning of the Mind Sight Program	31
Chapter 5	Laws and Principles of Mind Sight .	34
Chapter 6	Training Students in Mind Sight	39
Chapter 7	Advanced Exercises	51
Chapter 8	The Training Process	55
Chapter 9	To Be a Teacher	59
Chapter 10	Eva's Demonstration	67
Chapter 11	Students Discuss Mind Sight	70
Chapter 12	Practical Applications of Mind Sight	85
Chapter 13	Program for Advanced Research	90
Chapter 14	Mind Power Discovery	92
Chapter 15	Kirlian Photography	97
Chapter 16	Students to Remember	99
Chapter 17	Conclusion	106
Bibliography		108
Book Orders		109

Background Information

- By the Editor (Clear Springs Press)

Before the term "Remote View" entered our vocabulary and before there was any public awareness of the US Government Intelligence Agencies use of remote viewing as a means of gathering information, Lloyd Hopkins developed his Mind Sight training program. There is no relationship or connection between Mind Sight and Remote Viewing. They do of course access the same faculties of consciousness.

Lloyd Hopkins developed his mind sight training program with the intent of enabling the blind to see without the use of eyes. He gave numerous demonstrations before university groups and blind associations, etc. His students were mostly people who were sincere, free of skepticism and generally successful in their accomplishment of mind sight.

When Lloyd Hopkins passed this plane in 1994, no one continued his work. His mind sight program was not focused on self promotion and entertainment, but on training and empowering individuals to become greater people through developing their mind sight. That was more of a stretch of acceptance or more of a commitment of effort than most individuals could manage at that time. For the individuals involved, the mind sight training was an important chapter in their personal development. They all moved forward in pursuit of their own lives.

Lloyd Hopkins program was unique in several respects:

(1) Lloyd Hopkins did not charge for his training. His program was never an economic entity. This is in keeping with the Native American tradition that Spiritual gifts have to be gifted and cannot be sold. (Lloyd Hopking and some of his students were of Native American lineage.)

(2) Mr.Hopkins always instructed students one on one. He found this approach to be more effective than working with groups.

(3) His program was highly successful. Approximately 60% of his students were able to demonstrate some level of Mind Sight as a result of their training. 3% were exceptional and were able to do things like drive a car or read a book while blindfolded. I know of no other school or training program that can claim this kind of success.

(4) The Mind Sight program was focused on enabling an individual to develop the ability to exercise Mind Sight.

(5) He tailored the training to each individual. He would assess the mental, physical and energy status of his students and prescribe individual exercises for them based on the results of their tests.

(6) The "energy" status of the trainee was critical. Those with a high energy level were able to learn and perform and those with a low energy level could not. Mr. Hopkins used Kirlian photography to assess their energy level. This emphasis on energy is consistent with many shamanic and esoteric schools.

(7) Mr. Hopkins studied many Spiritual and esoteric traditions from many sources. He tied them all together with the principle of the three selves of the Huna as elaborated by Max Freedom Long.

(8) At some point in the training a distinct "breakthrough" was experienced where the student would begin literally seeing with their mind as if their mind had eyes of its own. Some reported a visual image of a television screen upon which they would literally "see" the object or scene of interest.

(9) The Mind Sight program was initially conceived as a practical application of enabling blind individuals to see without the use of their eyes. One of the star demonstrators of mind sight skills was, in fact, a blind person.

(10) It took approximately nine months to one year of persistent, consistent work to achieve success with an individual. Initially, training sessions were conducted one on one once per week. When the student's energy level was up to it, they would increase the number of sessions per week.

This manuscript contains the research done thus far regarding the visually handicapped by Lloyd F. Hopkins. There is no guarantee that the result of this work will provide all the scientific research answers. So Please accept this complimentary copy of Mind Sight and Perception. Perhaps your knowledge and expertise can help carry forward the effort begun here to improve the future for the visually handicapped and human kind.

God bless and help you
Lloyd F. Hopkins
Mind Sight and Perception
Research Center, Inc.
4015 255th St. East
Sanaway, WA 98387

(Note: This is Lloyd Hopkin's former address. It is no longer valid. Clear Springs Press is now the only source of this book.)

© 1988 by Lloyd Hopkins
Printed by Valley Press
Puyallup, Washington
Cover Photo by Bob Rudsit

© 2008 by Clear Springs Press, LLC

Clear Springs Press, LLC

http://www.clspress.com

Dedication

I dedicate this book to the many, many students, doctors, and scientists who encourage me to write an account of Mind Sight, so that millions may read, ponder, and explore the wonderful concept. Mind Sight could never have been a reality without the hard work, dedication, love and devotion of the students and all others involved.

To Drs. Theodore Smith and Henry Monteith, who gave me courage and inspiration. As scientists they encourage me to develop Mind Sight for demonstration purposes and arranged several demonstrations for us to build up our confidence.

To Dr. John Wilmarth for his 18 years of loyal friendship, input and advice.

To Dr. William Byers, an associate for the past 3½ years dedicated to the Development of Mind Sight.

To an unknown donor who believed in our work enough to support it for over a year.

All these have jointly brought this concept to the level of everlasting knowledge. Mind Sight lives today. Now!

When science can figure this all out, the world will also be indebted to you.

I Love you all.

(Lloyd Hopkins)

Foreword

Until the present time, men all over the world have believed that it is absolutely impossible to see without the aid of the eyes. However, if present investigators continue their work, this belief may be laid to rest.

In 1919, Dr. Nicola Tesla, the electrical engineering genius whose patents formed the foundation of the Westinghouse Corporation, described how he used "mind sight" to aid in his investigations. According to Tesla, he was able to "see" his inventions in his mind. He needed no models, drawings, or experiments, but was able to visualize a particular device with such facility that he could construct, test, and modify it totally in his mind without touching anything. Then when the device was perfected in his mind, he put it into concrete form, and it worked.

This process came to Tesla as a result of trying to deal with what he described as a boyhood affliction. This affliction was the periodic appearance of images, pictures, and scenes he imagined or other people had spoken of. Sometimes they were so powerful that he was unable to distinguish whether he was seeing a real object or just its image. Since the scenes were not always pleasant (a funeral, for instance), Tesla tried to control them or drive them out by concentrating on more desirable images. When he eventually ran out of familiar close-to-home objects and scenes to focus on, he became able to concentrate enough to start bringing in scenes from other places. Tesla claimed that he ultimately traveled to other cities and countries through his "mind sight."

In the 1930's, an East Indian magician named Kuda Bux performed amazing feats such as walking barefoot across burning coals heated to more than 800 degrees and allowing himself to be buried alive in a tightly filled grave for days at a time. Kuda Bux claimed that these "tricks" were made possible by the higher powers of the mind in which he had been trained since childhood. With various kinds of blindfolds, and once even after having a vision blurring drug put in his eyes by a doctor, Kuda Bux was able to "see" to read a variety of printed material put before him.

Neither of these men seemed to have made an effort to develop this mind sight in others, but limited themselves to experiments with their own minds. Now, however, Lloyd Hopkins of Tacoma, Washington, has been able to develop this ability in others. Thus far, he has trained more than thirty people to perform the feat.

Mr. Hopkins has been studying and experimenting in this area for approximately eighteen years. Though he is the first to admit that he has just barely opened the door to magnificent possibilities, he has developed a system of training that produces results. His students have demonstrated many times over the past several years before development and benefit of mankind, Mr. Hopkins has written this book to describe briefly what he has found and to present his ideas about how and why it works. This is a book of hope, faith, and confidence, and should be read by all those who believe in the development of their own minds and spirits.

Introduction by the Author

This book will present a concept that I hope you will find interesting and significant so that it will capture your attention and prompt you to study and action.

There are several groups of handicapped people; one of the most obvious is the blind. Society has established special schools to teach the blind special methods of reading, walking, and using guide dogs. Also, society provides a certain amount of academic and vocational skills needed to function with limited success in a world geared for sighted people. Blind people have advanced quite a bit from the days when they were almost completely dependent upon others for care and support.

However, service and training are still based on teaching the blind to accept a world of darkness and to feel their way through life. These blind people are still restricted in many ways. The things you and I take for granted – bright city lights, a beautiful sunset, the sight of their loved ones- are still denied to these people. They also are denied many jobs and numerous activities that the rest of us use to fill our lives.

These limitations I hope may not have to continue. In the past eighteen years of study and experimenting, I have come to believe that the blind may be taught to see through present investigation and continued research. In the past eighteen years I have taught many people of normal sight to see in varying degrees, with perception other than their eyes. During the past few years I have had success in working with some blind students. I am quite certain that more could learn to see.

Think for just a moment of the significance of this possibility: no more white canes, no more guide dogs, no more dependence on Braille, no more hesitant tentative steps while walking. Instead, blind people will have a chance at independence and fulfillment of life.

What I've just told you may sound unbelievable –like science fiction or wild dreams- but it is a reality. We have only scratched the surface in our study of this remarkable phenomena that I call "Mind Sight."

This book contains some of the findings of my eighteen-year journey into a realm that today is a normal part of my life. My experience and the demonstrations of my students prove how limitless the mind is once one determines to go beyond what is thought possible.

In this book I have tried to lay the ground work for those of you dedicated to humanitarian services or professional study. Teaching the blind to see was not my original intent; but during my course of research it was something that I brought to light and felt was something great that couldn't be ignored. The concept of Mind Sight is multi-faceted in which abilities are not restricted to just seeing without eyes. However, this book will concentrate on vision.

The material contained in this book is not all my own thought and words; much of it came from lectures, students, newspapers articles, and material read from books and other publications that I have gathered over the past eighteen years (the author of most of it unknown to me). I hope that by using a variety of sources I can put effectively into words the beliefs, ideas, principles, and philosophy that were necessary to mold Mind Sight into a proven and workable concept. I am grateful for the help that I received from the students, authors, and lectures.

The knowledge, secrets, and conditions necessary to allow an individual to avail himself to Mind Sight is all in the book and will come to you in the form of discussions and basic exercises. Read the material thoroughly. Any sentence, phrase, paragraph. Or series of paragraphs used more than once intentionally to emphasize its importance.

Please do not attempt to change the ideas, concepts, text, beliefs, principles, or philosophy, as well must be present for the concept to work.

Mind Sight, like other great mind advances, can be fully realized only by those who dedicate themselves and dare to think about and accept the unbelievable.

Lloyd F. Hopkins

Preface

The principle of Mind Sight is simple –**seeing without the use of one's eyes!** The concept of Mind Sight, however, is more complex. Live and videotaped demonstrations illustrate that blindfolded or blind, Mind Sight trainees can identify words, colors, and objects as well as read printed materials, all with 100 percent accuracy. Where does this skills come from? Who can learn it? How is it learned?

Current research into the function of the brain indicates that we typically use only 3% of our mind's capacity. Even Albert Einstein, one of our greatest geniuses, is estimated to have used only about 5% of the potential power of his mind. Researchers in the field of brain and mind functioning cannot account for the remainder of our mind's capacity.

We believe the skills taught in Mind Sight are part of this little exercised portion of the brain. The skills are available to all who are willing to take the time to learn to use them. Blind as well as sighted people can be taught Mind Sight skills. The only necessary aptitude seems to be the ability to believe that sightless vision is possible.

How is Mind sight learned? Through patience, perseverance, trial, and error, and a structured set of learned exercises that take the Mind Sight student from primary to advanced skills.

This book focuses on the development of the Mind Sight program and the steps involve in mastering a new skill – seeing without the use of one's eyes.

Chapter 1

A Demonstration

I was invited to give a demonstration and workshop of Mind Sight for the Regional Convention of The America Holistic Medical Association held in Seattle, Washington, April 5, 1986. The audience of psychiatrists, doctors, nurses, and visitors had no idea of what they were about to witness. Casual chatter filled the huge crowded room as I passed around the blindfolds to be used and asked the group to select one or two for student use. In this demonstration I used three students.

As the demonstration began, a sudden hush fell over the room. The first student to demonstrate was a registered nurse at a local hospital and had been a Mind Sight student for six months. The student demonstrated the ability to see objects and colored papers with the eyes firmly closed.

The second student, a Mind Sight student for one year, demonstrated the ability to see objects, white and colored papers completely blindfolded.

The third student named Deanna, a nurse, and a Mind Sight student for six years, gave an advanced demonstration. I adjusted the blindfold over Deanna's eyes, adding several folds of tissue underneath to make sure that no light could penetrate. I explained to the audience that the darker it was, the easier it would be for Deanna to see the pictures in her mind.

For the first demonstration, I set a color wheel with four colors –red, blue, green, and amber- on a card table and placed a chair about twenty feet away with its back to the wheel. Deanna sat down, blindfold in place, and proceeded to identify every color as I turned the wheel at random. The audience was intrigued. They had never seen a demonstration like this before, yet it was just the beginning of what we were to present.

For the next demonstration, a volunteer shuffled a deck of fifty cards consisting of colors and symbols, then placed the deck on the card table in the middle of the room. Deanna picked up the deck and identify every card in it without error in less than forty-five seconds.

To demonstrate Deanna's ability to identify spatial location, we asked a volunteer to put twenty papers – some white and some white with red print- in a wide circle on the floor. After Deanna walked around the circle and identified each paper's color and spatial orientation, the volunteer was asked to place solid colored papers over each of the papers on the floor. Again, Deanna identified each of the papers as she walked around the circle.

By this time, the Mind Sight demonstration had completely captures the audience's attention. The room grew very quiet. What would happen next? Deanna took a deck of regular playing cards from a volunteer and separated them into suits in less than forty seconds, without error. She then quickly went though a deck of sixty-five cards of pictures, numbers and colors, identifying them all. The audience broke into applause and some observers took notes, jotting down questions and discussing the demonstration with co-workers. The excitement was building.

The demonstration were even more impressive. From a box of flash math cards, I began flashing arithmetic problems in front of Deanna. As quickly as I showed the card, she read each problem and gave the correct solution. However, the most incredible display was to come.

A large table was cleared and brought to the center of the room, and I then asked the audience to bring some personal articles, such as rings, money, watches, cards, and photos, to the table. Deanna walked around the table and identified all articles to the satisfaction of owners. Again, for the final demonstration, Deanna read several pieces of printed material, including cards, bulletins, letters, and from a short handbook. She read it all, out loud, never missing a word.

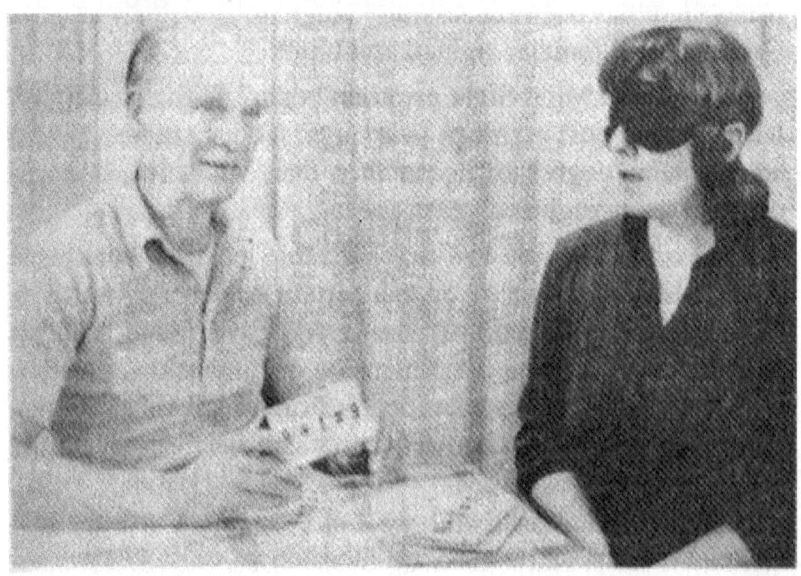

Lloyd Hopkins flips through a deck of long division flash cards as a thoroughly blindfolded Deanna Calef gives the correct answer.

As was typical of over hundred demonstrations we have given, we were immediately besieged with compliments and questions. What had happened here? Was it magic? No, there was no special equipment needed, no preparation time, no tricks. Was it psychic? No, psychic have been unable to demonstrate, on demand and with 100 percent accuracy the abilities of a student of Mind Sight. Is Deanna gifted in some special way? No, no more than any other human being on this earth. Deanna had simply learned a set of skills that can be taught to anyone with faith, perseverance, and an open mind. Mind Sight has been successfully taught to students young and old, male and female, sight and blind.

How did the Mind Sight program begin? With curiosity and with vision... just eighteen years ago. Today, there seems to be a grater degree of acceptance than when I first started demonstrating eighteen years ago.

Professional people are making more positive comments. After a demonstration given at a certain university, one of the professors commented, "It seems you have found a way to pass back and forth into a dimension or dimensions unknown at present." After another demonstration given to a small group, a psychologist after witnessing the demonstration given by a lady blind from birth, he said, "I couldn't for a moment understand it. Only a fool could deny what I saw. Hopkins has tapped a whole dimension of existence we can hardly comprehend." And, after a demonstration to a medical group, an observer stated, "Watching the demonstration was like watching science fiction. Hopkins is ahead of his time." A milder comment was made by a scientist after watching a demonstration given at his university: "I am baffled, to say the least."

After giving many demonstrations to psychology classes conducted by Dr. Jessie Nolph at Pacific Lutheran University, Dr. Nolph remarked one day that student acceptance of Mind Sight has risen from about 15 percent to 85 percent, which gives a vote of confidence to our effort.

Chapter 2

Mind Sight. What is it?

Mind Sight. What is it? Where does it come from? How does it work? What are its practical applications? How is it observed? What are the future research possibilities of Mind Sight? In my eighteen years of demonstrating the physical potential for Mind Sight, these questions have been more frequently asked after each demonstration.

Mind Sight is a term I used to label the phenomenon that I discovered come eighteen years ago. Though, not I nor anyone else can totally explain it at this time, I will answer these questions to the best of my ability throughout the book.

Mind Sight and Perception is, I believe a science that allows man to learn to integrate mind, body, and soul to form a power of perception both internally and externally that is in accordance with his creative inheritance, and to use this inherent power to see without eyes and increase awareness beyond known limitations. The Science of Mind Sight and Perception is based upon ascertained and verified facts, and upon phenomena that are obtained through observation and mental and physical experiences, and aided by inductive and synthentical analogy. In other words, the practice and principles of Mind Sight are in perfect harmony with the highest human potential and principles of science.

THE CENTER

The Mind Sight Center is a tax exempt corporation engaged in a humanitarian activity that is different from any other in this country. The center is engaged in both research and training. Through the research that has been completed, we are able to train teachers to see without the use of their eyes, so that they, in turn, may train the visually handicapped to perceive objects and colors, to walk unaided in unfamiliar surroundings, and to read printed material. This is not done through the use of Braille, canes, guide dogs, or other commonly used methods of assisting the blind; it is done by the use of senses not normally exercised. The training process takes roughly nine months to a year or more, depending on the condition of the individual. People blind from birth, as well as those who are blind as a result of accidents or disease, have been successfully trained by the center, and the evidence is available to anyone who may be interested.

Medical doctors, psychologists, nurses, and other professional and lay people who are not visually handicapped have learned these skills while blindfolded to prove to themselves that Mind Sight is a reality, and to give aid in this work. Those proficient in Mind Sight are convinced that this is not just mumbo jumbo used to extract money from the public. There is no charge for the many demonstrations that have been given in colleges, service clubs, and on television shows.

Advanced research in the field of mind perception reveals that the human being possesses abilities that ha or she has either forgotten how to use or has not developed due to lack of necessity. Research will continue to improve our teaching techniques so that the center will be able to reach more people. At present, each student attends a two-hour session each week. As students are taught on a one-to-one basis, more teachers are needed.

Mind Sight is multifaceted –abilities are not restricted to just seeing without eyes- however, as the concept is still new and not yet widely accepted or heard of, this book will concentrate on the visual aspect to conserve the research, teaching principles and progress that have been made in these areas, and hopefully, to interest others in continuing the work that I have started. We have only touched the surface of this thing. Much more research is required, and the more minds that are put to this task, the faster people can be helped through the application el Mind Sight. Undisputedly, teaching the blind to see is one of the greatest rewards in the work that I have accomplished.

Mind Sight is not respecter of persons; young and old, men and women, sighted or blind are all eligible to learn, as it is evident that this phenomena is part of everyone's physiological make up. The result that each student experiences vary according to the time that they devote to learning. Some people learn faster than others, just as some people run faster than others. However, except in the most exceptional of cases, most can achieve results if even not at the same time.

Until vary recently, I had been unable to find any mention of discoveries even remotely related to Mind Sight. The only book written about similar research was that of French scientist and author, Jules Romains. A PhD in physiology and botany, he did research sixty-five years ago and published his book in French. It was translated into English in 1977, seven years after I had discovered Mind Sight. His book, *Eyeless Sight*, explains that he did not know how the phenomenon actually worked, although he made some conjectures about it and proceeded to leave it up to future research to explain what actually takes place. I am repeating this effort; I shall continue to apply Mind Sight and research further uses and applications.

Herein plans for technical instruction in Mind Sight and specific procedures relating to personal work are contained. I am offering a general, technical and non-technical survey of the principles, laws and methods I used to gain and understand Mind Sight. This book is not intended for the scientist of profession only, but for all who are willing to open their minds and dedicate the time and effort necessary for this method of eyeless vision to be used.

This book and facts about my learning, teaching and living Mind Sight are true.

The truth of Mind Sight, as we have demonstrated over a hundred times to universities, scientific communities, doctors, psycho-gists, and visual professionals (not to mention magicians!), has contradicted many theories about the nature of thought and logic. Scientists tell me that I have stumbled upon the fringes of a new truth that could have value beyond any measure in science, education, and medicine; there are now more hope and possibilities for the handicapped, as well as possibilities for further development of human mind.

Experiences that are uncommon are especially difficult to relate to in written form. What can be read here is only a glimpse of what can be achieved or even imagined. Explore this new concept with an open mind, and perhaps Mind Sight will be part of your life.

Currently, the Center is operating on part-time basis. It is limited by a lack of facilities and the financial strain of providing equipment for a higher degree of monitoring. There are now over forty people who wish to begin training that we do not have time for, as well as over 85,000 visually handicapped in this country who could benefit from this training, including 14,000 in Washington.

This book is in part offered as a fund raising effort to ask for assistance in a humanitarian way that is unique: with Mind Sight the blind may be taught to perceive their environment in a manner that has never before been achieved and they may be able to realize their full potential. I hope to ensure that this potential is not lost to the world.

We invite and welcome challenges by scientists, psychologists, physicians, and others to see the results of our work and to visit our center at their convenience for a demonstration.

Chapter 3

A Research Project
In Human Behavior

I wish to impress upon the reader that the mere act of reading this book is not likely to do much in the direction of self-improvement. But the complete understanding and application of the principles, rules, and discipline taught here will –according to the degree of attention and acceptance brought a mew world of wonder.

Before my interest in mind and the discovery of Mind Sight, I had little or no faith in the possibility of any person being able to recondition his mind and inner self to the degree of reading a book without eyes or the possibility of teaching others this respect. The person making such a claim two hundred years ago would in all probability have been treated as a witch and burned at the stack. I wouldn't be at all surprised if my statements in this book are questioned by some; but this great discovery may someday be held dear to the millions of people who have a strong desire to comprehend the power of the mind. This is proven by the great value human being place upon knowing one's self. Yet how little the real science of mind is understood by the scientists today. But great strides are started in this direction.

One of the first obstacles that science must overcome is that there is yet no way to make some philosophies practical, because there are no fixed rules for determining whether a man is endowed with god-like abilities. The science of Mind sight, when fully understood, could perhaps explain the great points of diversity found in man's whole nature. And furthermore, I hope that Mind Sight will explain, as has yet no other science, the only practical way to man's perfection and reality in our Creator. How much of the Creator is in us? How much of us is in the Creator?

No science has been able to give a complete analysis of our mental faculties and to answer the great number of questions about man. It is my sincere hope that Mind Sight will enlighten science in this endeavor.

The next statement I make with tongue in cheek, because I have a very dear friend who is a blind physiologist and we have talked along these lines several times. It would seem the modern aspect of physiological research in relation to the localization of centers of ideation and motion in the brain seems most conclusive. But what of Mind Sight? In my research with individual students I sometimes am led to believe that there is no specific brain center for eyeless sight or Mind Sight. It seems this sight is resident in man only through certain beliefs, faith, and discipline, not in any specific cerebral center, and can be understood only through the very nature of man's creation.

The organic remains of the earliest type of human species that have been found demonstrate to some scientists that man started life comparatively a child in mental powers and knowledge. With all the faculties that humans now possesses, we have power to choose, according to likes and dislikes and judgment. We are also endowed with the ability to learn from experience and reflection, without any good or evil in our nature.

Historical evidence seems to show that all humans were first governed mainly through power of self-preservation, combined with the objective perception and domestic faculties. At that time his superior faculties must have been feeble. Over the centuries of man's climb through evolution, today we from birth have a great deal of capability and we must simply realize what we already know. That is why education is so important –to bring out the unused or unknown knowledge.

I have noticed as I continue in my education that I am now more selective and I don't absorb everything. I pick and choose things that are necessary to my work. Now my mind seems to direct me to the right things and just leaves the rest alone. It is not that I don't know that other things exist, but they aren't necessary for my existence or pattern of life. To me, they are like untruths (they could be true to someone else, though). I must know that they do exist in order to discriminate between the truths and the untruths. But I still have the ability to choose that which will challenge my reasoning to benefit my work.

I cannot help but think that some of the abilities in Mind Sight came about from a result of the many books I read. It was not really what I read but how I interpreted it, how my mind perceived it, and how often times it would seem that I had lived the words at another time. I can't help but think this technique could have been used thousands of years ago. Years ago, perhaps Mind Sight was common knowledge. Then new technology made things too easy, the mind became lazy, and the whole concept was lost or traded off for something requiring less mental dexterity. Some time ago I read a book *Love and Wisdom*, by Richard Hubler, who apparently had some thought along these lines when he wrote about "the loss of the mystical power of speech. In the days of Samuel, words had tremendous forces, far beyond their meaning. They might heal, excite, fury, or tame passion, even perform miracles at the intonation of certain phrases. Force sprang out of syllables describing an object with almost the power within the object itself. Cussing, you may imagine, was a fatal talent; just as blessing was a high and joyful one. The ear and the tongue were fearful weapons together. Now the are edgeless and rusty, no more than the gobble of geese or the grunting of an animal."

Max Freedom Long, in his book, *Secrets of Science Behind Miracles*, tells of his first visit with Dr. William Tufts Brigham, curator for the Bishop Museum in Honolulu, Hawaii. He had heard that the doctor spent many years delving into Hawaiian things, and hoped he could find the true answer regarding the phenomenal abilities of the Kahunas (priests) of Hawaiian people. Dr. Brigham listened to questions for some time and then answered:

> "For forty years I have been studying the Kahunas to find out the answer to the questions you have asked. The Kahunas do use what you have called magic. They do heal, they do kill, they do look into the future and change it fir their clients. Many were impostors, but some were genuine. Some even used this magic to fire walk over and across lava overflows barely cooled enough to carry the weight of a man. I have been trying for forty years to answer this questions for myself –wuthout success."

Dr. Brigham told of other abilities ha had researched such as the power of vital force, the Kahuna psychology, the ten elements of the ancient Huna system, instant healing, raising the dead, controlling winds and weather, and many more feats in mind control. Many of these feats I learned and used in some of my power of the mind demonstrations. To me this was common knowledge, apparently I had used these abilities before.

After the discovery of the islands by Captain Cook, he wrote fantastic stories about the Kahuna powers. The missionaries began coming to the islands thinking that they must save these poor wretched people and that only Christ could perform such miracles. Most of these powers were stamped out with the take over of the islands by the white man's religion. Little did the missionaries know that they destroyed great mental feats in the name of Christianity.

Chapter 4

The Beginning of The Mind Sight Program

In 1968 started Roy Forest Products Company in Roy, Washington. About a year later, I found that I had a serious heart condition and I realized I needed to find something to do with my time that would excite me mentally but not physically. My search was born.

Earlier I had read *The Secret Science Behind Miracles*, by Max Freedom Long. I was challenged to do some research on the principles of parapsychology, to satisfy my own curiosity. In 1970 I opened and office, Parapsychology Research, and ran an ad in the paper inviting people to volunteer to participate in a variety of experiments. My goal was to form a strong enough hypothesis to enable continuing research. I explore all available avenues of knowledge, including hypnosis, psychometric analysis, clairvo-yance, psychokinesis, levitation, mental telepathy, and astral projection. Each has some validity, but they are elementary abilities when compared or contrasted with Mind Sight as we know it today.

Historically. Precedents for eyeless sight abound. One story, in particular, prompted my thirst for more knowledge in this area. I read in the newspaper about a man in Greece who claimed that, "Many, many years ago many people were ship watchers. These people were designed to keep an eye on the horizon and to notify the authorities when a shop came over the horizon. These people got so they could identify and see a ship far before it reaches the horizon." Was this ability inherited? Psychic? Teachable? I had to find out!

After several months of experimenting with volunteers and with myself as chief guinea pig, there was no way I could actually document or validate sight without eyes. Yet in history these skills or gifts were occasionally demonstrable. What was the key?

I realized that I had been using the same assumptions as other researchers, which led me, as well as them, to no physical proof. I discovered I was thinking in a restricted area. How could I evaluate fairly the theories and results when my thinking was limited? Traditional tests and results from out-of-body experiences, extrasensory perception, and clairvoyance did not yield the results I was looking for –100 percent accuracy.

I discovered that I had to challenge all other thinking as well as authority, religion, and science. I had to re-examine my own mind in its entirety –my faith, beliefs, ideas, and concepts. I had to create from my discoveries and offer the world a physical truth –a reality.

As my faith and beliefs became stronger, some of the pieces of the puzzle began to come together. One of the first things I discovered was that no one factor could stand alone. The approach must be made by using the combined energies of the mind, both physical and spiritual. The student must rely not on meditation, as I had been doing, but on intense concentration. Sometimes I would concentrate so hard that I was sure my brain would burst. One of my students later explained to a reporter, "I feel I have worked every atom in my body."

Through study of laws of the mind, spiritual principles, and physical faculties, the Mind Sight program evolved. There were setbacks that frustrated me and delayed progress for months, but then there were astounding advances that encouraged me to follow the path I had set for myself.

At first, it was a monumental task to apply the various factors and exercises into a workable concept. I would end up far away from my goal with no place to go. Finally, my mind started to see flashes and pictures as a sign for motion. I began to think of these flashes and pictures without meaning. But motion representing what? After several months of trial and error, I developed another principle to put motion into play, with psycho-physical skills still the governing factor. Something was still missing. Bit by bit, I pieced together a format to lead the mind of the student to accept its inherent potential.

Today, Mind sight is a reality. Any student who will believe, study, and persevere, and who will not be afraid of hard work, can achieve 100 percent accuracy in seeing without eyes.

How does this happen? Where would you begin as a Mind Sight student?

Chapter 5

Laws and Principles of Mind Sight

Mind Sight exercises have been carefully developed to make use of as many faculties of the human mind as possible. The exercises are designed to cause the mind to open up and respond to the factors created by the exercise, to hold the attention to the goal, and to increase the power of will and mind. These are what I call "psycho-physical" skills.

My research has proved that we can expand our mental power if we take the time and effort necessary to concentrate on six most important factors: purpose, desire, will, concentration, truth, and faith. That is, you begin with a *purpose* or goal; then you must have the *desire* to fulfill it. You must use your *will* to put your mind in motion and *concentrate* harder than you ever have in your life. To accomplish this expanded awareness, it is necessary to start with the smallest *truth* and then build toward greater truths. Finally, you must believe completely and have *faith* in your Creator, in what you are doing, in yourself as part of your Creator, and in your Creator as part of yourself.

Of the many laws and principles involved in the perfection of Mind Sight, one factor in particular was important in helping me understand the concept. This principle is continuous and intelligent thought about the growth of any mental power. With certain regulated exercises, this positive power can be applied to enhance the learning of Mind Sight. These exercises must be carefully worked out to help the student's mind to open up and respond to the factors created by the exercise, to hold the attention to the desired goal, and to increase the power of will and mind. I call these psycho-physical skills.

Psycho-physical skills are governed by their own laws, discovered by people who wish or dare to reach certain goals, such as playing the piano or singing, and who have attained, as a result of hard work, long practice and patience, their desired results. The exercises needed to attain these skills had to be constructed to contain other factors such as faith, truth, impressions, memory, will, vital force, association, and perception. Perception –the mind's ability to see things as the are- must be a conscious effort. Few people pay enough attention to their senses to employ them thoroughly or intelligently. I found that perception is absolutely necessary, and complete concentration on an article such as a ball, color wheel, or paper will increase control of the mind to an astonish degree.

People are capable of a thousand forms of action that are taken for granted. In Mind Sight, certain progressive faculties must be observed, especially when we are working with students who are blind or going blind. These faculties are what give us the capability to perceive the color, quality, relative size, and configuration, of material objects; active focus on these faculties gives us practical experience in controlling the mind.

The mind and brain contain a multitude of powers or agencies such as intellect, will, judgment, and attentiveness, that produce mental activities. The mind and brain control the emotional system the same way they control behavioral activities and. Like everything else in the emotional system, they must reach a balance with all other human factors to result in the fullest restoration of health. The following faculties are woven into the exercises Min Sight students experience at each level of their training.

- Coloration: Along with association, coloration gives perception of color –the power to perceive qualities, shades, tints, hues; the capacity to reproduce, mingle, and blend colors; And, for those going blind, memory of colors.

- Gravitation: Allows perception such as touch, the power to perceive force and resistance, and the ability to balance muscular locomotion un harmony with gravitation.

- Size: Enables perception of the relative size of different objects and their relative proportions such as length, depth, and breadth. It also allows judgment of the weight and strength of various objects by their relative size.

- Configuration: Enables us to distinguish between the various configurations in nature –the difference in faces, pictures, outlines, and shapes- and the capacity to reproduce different configurations according to a given model. This faculty is vital in teaching students blind from birth.

- Expressions: Enables us to express our thoughts and emotions by words. This faculty is common to all teachers and is also especially important for the blind student.

- Order: Gives perception of details, the ability to ascertain particulars and work by rule and system, and the tendency to be orderly. It provides the desire to have a place in the memory bank for specific knowledge to draw upon when needed.

- Acoustiveness: Allows us to remember sounds, to perceive distant sounds and different voices, and to sense emphasis and pronunciation. Some blind students excel in this faculty but, oddly, the majority do not.

- Observation: enable us to observe different objects as having separated existence regardless of their proportions or their qualities. This faculty provides the tendency to focus the objective faculties on any concrete object or abstract idea that may demand current attention. It also includes the desire to obtain knowledge by observing and gathering facts, and the power to retain facts.

- Discrimination: Allows students to dissociate phenomena and abstract ideas and to perceive incongruities, defects, and false analogies. This faculty gives students the power of rapid criticism and the ability to expose error.

- Locomotion: Enables students to discern localities, to locate new places, and to accommodate to new localities.

- Causativeness: Enables students to analyze and clarify phenomena and abstract ideas, to understand various concepts, to ascertain the first principle of a concept or subject, to resolve abstract ideas into practical applications, and to do analytical analysis as opposed to synthesis.

- Analogy: Allows students to perceive similarities in the repetition of phenomena and abstract ideas, to perceive resemblances and reason by induction and perception of analogies and harmonies, to perceive truths that are not known, and to combine and form complex ideas from simple ones.

- Prescientiousness: gives students the power to look ahead, perceive a concept, and put it to practical use to forecast the future.

These faculties are all vital and are interwoven into Mind Sight training exercises. However, many other factors are combined into the training. I find that new methods of relaxing while practicing deep concentration must also be used. These methods must be assigned by the teacher rather than decide upon individually by the student. Students must practice awareness outside of sessions with the teacher, and must maintain a conscious will in all activities. The confident expectation of success is indispensable to the achievement of Mind Sight. The positive mind demands and achieves the things it wants; students must repeatedly impress upon their minds the desire to accomplish Mind Sight. Memory is a vital factor for students who are going blind or who are born blind; in fact, the success or failure of a student can greatly depend on the ability to retain and recall ideas, principles, thoughts, observations, or reflections. The power of will is another important component; discipline of one's will is essential to success in Mind Sight.

Mind Sight can be neither bought nor sold. It is given as a gift of love to the trainee from the trainer, and each is the beneficiary. Should a trainee attempt to pay for the training, the bond is broken or lost, because the student feels he is "buying" and open mind. The student's commitment to the training, and to key to successful Mind Sight training.

Chapter 6

Training Students in Mind Sight

The student should not be concerned when he or she makes a mistake, as this is commonplace. Although each mistake is corrected, the reason for the error is that objects bring awareness in different ways and at different times, and some days you will not be able to do as well as you did previously. It is only natural that when your mind accepts the idea that you can do these things, more rapid progress will take place.

Students are told that they will learn through repetition and psycho-physical skills, along with other factors –faith, belief, truth, concentration- and that they must be corrected each time an error is made. Each time the student makes a mistake, he or she must attempt to see the object in its correct appearance and its correct location. The mind is stubborn. It doesn't readily accept the idea that one really wants to do these things in this manner, and it must be convinced that one really does want to do this before it begins to cooperate.

While attempting the various exercises involved, there is a great tendency for the mind to become bored. It is important to know just how long to keep at an exercise before it is overdone. This is an important skill that a teacher must have, because each student progress differently. Thus, only an experienced teacher may accomplish this task. Additionally, it is exceeding important that the student follows directions and that he or she not try to use his own ideas of how to learn this skills. This is one of the two places where learning can be stifled, the other being not finishing the course after it is started. This is the reason that there is no homework in lessons, although there are some extra studies in which exercises are assigned. The weekly lessons resemble music lessons, but there are no scales to take home to practice. It is possible to miss some lessons and continue, but the learning process is only prolonged.

It appears to be easier for a woman to learn these skills than for a man and children can be taught more easily than adults. Knowing this, one can readily appreciate that adults have a more difficult time in opening up their minds and freeing themselves from preconceived ideas. Men have sometimes found it hard to accept that women can learn to do this more easily than they.

There are nine devices used in training:
1. Balls
2. Color Wheel
3. Cards
4. Tapes
5. Papers –white or with red print
6. Colored Papers
7. Eye Mask
8. Light Projector
9. Reading Material

Before I discuss the exercise step-by-step, I would like the reader to consider again that there are several principles, laws and disciplines involved in Mind Sight. However, there is one outstanding principle that is an important factor in helping me to understand and find a key to Mind Sight –certain regulated exercises influence the function itself. These exercises have to be carefully worked out to cause the mind to open up, to hold the attention to the desired goal, and to increase the power of will and mind. These are called psycho-physical skills. These psycho-physical skills are governed by their own laws that have been discovered and utilized by people who acquire certain skills, such as playing the piano or singing. There are ultimately forty-two steps in the process of attaining Mind Sight.

You will eventually understand more about the importance of understanding human nature –the emotions, instincts, and reasoning faculties of man- through your ability to use Mind Sight effectively under all sort of conditions. This ability will grow in proportion to your knowledge of how one mind influences another.

This information will be given for your encouragement and understanding, to educate you concerning the presence of certain laws, principles , and faculties, and to show the road on which you are about to travel. I don't intend to provide at this time until the study of Mind Sight is complete.

TRAINING BEGINS

As a volunteer in the training program of Mind Sight, you will begin your training immediately as follows:

1. A Kirlian Test: The instructor uses special Kirlian photographic equipment to take slides of the student's fingertips. Certain physical and emotional levels are detected through colors and patterns that appear after development of the film. This is a helpful part of gauging the pace at which the instructor designs exercises suited to each student's particular needs.
2. Psychic Test: On such a test, the instructor holds up cards unrevealed to the student

as he writes down which color or symbol the card contains.

3. A Comprehension Test: This is a test containing sentences stem concerning one's feeling about different things; it is a typical psychological evaluation. An example is "the student completes each stem."

4. The student is shown video recordings of other students during their training and will listen to some tapes. He or she is then introduced to the teacher, who instruct him to observe, listen to, and study other information presented.

Several of the beginning exercises or steps are then shown and explained. During all of this, the student is evaluated by the teacher regarding interest show and comprehension expressed.

During early discussions between student and teacher, the teacher's prime task is to work through any student indifference, resistance, or antagonism immediately by showing and explaining to the student the advantages to be gained by listening and observing . The student is then scheduled for a specific day and hour of the week for continued training. He or she is also advised about certain things that enter into our lives that can at times upset the best laid plans and create absolutely unforeseen situations. Sometimes these situations can be avoided by looking ahead a little and conducting open discussions. The student's desire to committing to weekly training is a requirement that is emphasized.

THE EXERCISE

As you are introduced to the various steps or exercises, all the principles and factors needed to open the mind's visual field and set the goal are models into easy-to-follow steps. I will explain a few.

Magnetic Attraction is one of the first exercises. The student is asked to stand in the center of the room with hands clasped in a prayer like position and eyes closed. The instructor asks the student to keep the hands pointed as the teacher walks around. The student is instructed to pay attention to what is sensed. As the teacher stops with arms extended toward the student, hands held in an open position, the student tries to place his or her hands into the opening of the teacher's hands. If the student feels he or she has done this, the hands are opened to reveal the truth. In time, the perimeter of the teacher's changes from small to large. As the student improves, he or she is able to point to the position of the teacher with 100 percent accuracy. This exercise is geared to give the student certain positive feed back and to verify the truth so that the student's mind can accept that which is going on as a reality. The reality, in turn gives faith, trust, will, and confidence.

Next, there are several motions exercises. The student is asked to stand about twenty feet from the teacher. With the student's eyes open, the teacher explains the exercise. The teacher signals for the student to come forward, the teacher puts his hands in a stop position. The student is instructed to stop about thirty inches from the teacher in order to avoid any physical contact. He or she motions for the student to back up until the starting point is reached. The teacher then motions the student to turn to the right and left and make c complete 360 degree circle in both directions, and then a stop signal is given. The student is then mentioned to bend down at the knees and then to stand erect. In addition to the hand motion, each student is asked to listen for mental commands to each motion. This enables the mind and body to learn to perform in unity. During the exercise, the teacher watches the student closely to see if there may be an equilibrium problem. If not, the student is then asked to close the eyes, and the exercise is repeated at least three times each session. Many times the student experiences a balance problem during the first two or three tries, but it soon disappear. If the problem does not disappear the student is then given another test – to walk a line. This test is similar to the one the state patrol gives drivers possibly under the influence of alcohol. This test usually corrects any problem.

In another motion exercise the student, still standing about twenty feet from the teacher, is asked to open the eyes. The teacher stands against an object or in front of an object such as a door and then comes toward the student with hands in motion likened to a windshield wiper. When the teacher reaches approximately eighteen inches of the student, he or she waves the hands on the left and right sides of the student, then front and back , back and top, top and front, front and back, and sides again. The teacher then moves back to the starting point. The exercise is repeated with the student's eyes closed. Standing in front of an object (door or wall), the teacher asks the student to envision him or her standing there. Of course the student is then compelled to use a little imagination to envision the teacher at the object. The teacher asks the student to continue to envision him or her as he or she walks toward the student and to envision the motion of the teacher's arms and hands around the student's body. As the teacher backs away, the student is instructed to try to hold a picture of the motion in mind until the teacher reaches the starting point. This exercise is repeated at least three times each session.

These exercises are very important, especially to the blind. They open the mind to envision objects and motion at different distances and at different levels. You would be surprised how quickly this exercise will produce results. Not only will the blind person become aware of the motion, but he or she will soon be able to see both the teacher's and his or her own hands. The student is directed in many kinds of motion so that when a motion crosses the visual field of the mind, the mind will be able to see and discern the difference between moving and inanimate.

THE COLOR WHEEL

The student sits in chair about ten feet in front of a color wheel, back to the wheel or light. The wheel has four basic colors: red, blue, green, and amber.

In this exercise, the student closes the eyes, and the teacher turns on the light of the color wheel. The student rolls up the sleeves and turns in the collar of his or her shirt, in order to have as much uncovered flesh as possible. This is to acquaint the student with opening all channels of sensitivity and receptivity while trying to see the colors. The student is instructed as follow: "This color is red; allow this color to bathe the exposed part of the body so that mind and body will know, accept, and recognize this color when it appears again as red." The remaining colors on the wheel are explained to the student in the same manner so that the mind and body will begin to recognize each as such. Since a student who has been blind from birth cannot recognize these colors and has no knowledge of color, he or she is instructed to use an association, such as an emotion or feeling, to identify with the color.

Each color emanating from the color wheel is described as a live or penetrating color. This association sets up flashes and patches of individual colors in the student's visual field. Later, the colors are associated with objects.

THE BALLS

Exercise 1: In this exercise, a nine-inch plastic ball is used. The ball is thrown to the student (whose eyes are closed) to catch directly or as it bounces from the floor. This action will eventually travel across the visual field of the student's mind as dimension, color, and motion. It will heighten the reflexes by the speed or velocity of the traveling ball.

Exercise 2: In this exercise, a large beach ball with at least six colors is used. The mind of the student starts to pick up colors as they appear on the ball and becomes more aware of colors flashes as the ball travels back and forth from teacher to student. When the ball is held in the student's hand, the student must learn to point out individual colors from the group of colors.

THE CENTER ATTRACTION EXERCISE

This exercise uses white papers with memo printing and white papers with red pictures that are placed upon the floor. The student is led past the papers and focuses upon each one individually as an object. Once the object is accepted by the mind, the mind sets into motion a specific action to evaluate the object as to color, location, orientation, and dimension.

COLORED PAPERS

In this exercise papers of fifteen different colors are used. Everything seen with normal vision or memory vision has color in some way. After the student is able to envision the various colors individually, the colored papers are placed upon the white papers to offer a color contrast. The white paper and color contrasts are stored in the mind for future reference and association with other objects.

Another exercise with colored papers is done sitting at a table; the instructor names the color of each paper while the blindfolded student is instructed to visualize these. The papers are named repeatedly backward and forward until the student is confident of recognizing the colors. Then the papers are shuffled, and the student attempts once again to identify them. This exercise is one of the first used. When the student seems to be fairly proficient, the colored papers on the floor are used as described above.

READING LETTERS

To begin to learn to read letters, the student sits in front of an eye chart. He or she is told what the letters in each line are and attempt to magnify these letters in the mind to a size that would fill an advertising billboard. This exercise is continued until the student feels able to do it. The exercise is not prolonged but is repeated almost every week.

MENTAL PICTURES OR IMAGERY EXERCISES

In developing power of effective imagery nothing is too trivial. In our training a student is asked to look at the face of the teacher; when the image is fixed in the student's mind the student will close his or her eyes and raise the right forefinger. When the image starts to fade the student raise the left forefinger and open the eyes to renew the mental image. At first, the student time of holding an image is approximately fifteen seconds, but through practice the time can be extended to twenty hours or more. With more picture and image practice trials, the student will begin to remember every detail; The more complete the picture and the detail, the higher the consistency. When reading a book or explaining details in a picture while blindfolded, it is necessary that effort be perfected.

It is important to emphasize that each exercise is repeated weekly, and that continual feedback by the teacher is vital. Each incorrect guess must be corrected immediately, and the teacher must be able to judge each student's individual attention span and willpower. These exercises are repeated periodically throughout the training period.

You have undoubtedly discovered by experience that that which is worthwhile is not accomplished easily, but this doesn't mean that it is impossible. It can be done, and you can do it. Persons who have experienced accomplishment in this manner have admitted that their results and transitions were almost unbelievable. The path to Mind Sight is more easily traveled than imagined if one is willing to complete the journey and accept the fact that obstacles and problems encountered can be overcome. There are benefits to be gained immediately, and many will experience long-range effects as well.

There are no magical words or spell that give a person Mind Sight. No amount of exercises or drills can induce this process without expert help. The teacher explains to the student why, especially at first, it is necessary to follow strict instructions and will prescribe the necessary exercises that will lift morale and contribute to an atmosphere of success. A hands-on experience of watching Mind Sight demonstrated by an accomplished student provides the stimulus for belief in one's own potential. Encouraged by the teacher every step of the way, the student will perceive and accept continued progress. Without this there is no way to build or measure the truth. If one comes into this discipline in any way insecure or unsure of himself or herself, continued practice with Mind Sight techniques is bound to build confidence and faith, especially as sightless vision is achieved.

    I recall a particular lady who, because of her mental and physical condition (she was blind), was very insecure. After attending a Mind Sight demonstration she asked me if I could help her in the use of Mind Sight. After working with this lady for several weeks I saw her progress becoming slower and slower because of negative influence in her home and from other people. I told her straight forward that unless she prescribed to the faith and confidence necessary to lift her morale and contribute to an atmosphere of positive success that she would be wasting her time as well as mine. Tears filled her eyes as she told me she would try harder to believe in her own potential. I assigned her exercise time with an advanced student. Within three months she made a remarkable change in her attitude and accomplishment. It was competitiveness that turned the tide of her thinking. "If the advanced student can do it, so can I." This woman went on to become one of my best students and advanced into achievements beyond her wildest dreams.

Chapter 7

Advanced Exercises

After the student has gained 100 percent proficiency en the basic exercises described in Chapter 6, more advanced exercises are introduced. (Blindfold is used.)

>Learns to read the ophthalmoscope.
>Learns to read cards, symbols, color.
>Learns to read printed material / books.
>Learns to expand his visual field to 360°.
>Learns to project the mind with 100 percent accuracy to greater distances.

The Ophthalmoscope: This instrument was originally used by optometrists and ophthalmologists. It allows viewing slides of letters, symbols, and pictures. A large symbol made up of lines like a letter T is rotated around a clock face and the student is eventually able to see these symbols projected on a movie screen in a dark room. Sometimes red and green colors are used as an overlay. Also, letters are projected on the screen –sometimes plain white, sometimes red and green mixed, or full red or green covering letters and symbols. This exercise is repeated in succeeding weeks until the student is able to read with 100 percent accuracy.

Cards and Symbol Exercise: After the student has gained proficiency in the above exercise (usually in about six months) he sits at a table and a deck of cards is placed on the table. This deck contains twenty-five cards of five symbols: a triangle, an arrow, a check mark, four dots, and a heart. These are all printed in black ink on a white background. The instructor places the cards one at a time in front of the blind or blindfolded student and names each one. Each subsequent card is placed on top of the previous card and identified for the student. Training on the ophthalmoscope has prepared the student to learn to do this without much trouble. Later, the cards are shuffled and the student attempts to identify each card as it is placed in front of him or her. If an error is made the instructor corrects it and waits until the student actually sees the card before going to the next card. The first time the student correctly sees and identify all twenty-five cards is an exciting experience.

Color Cards: This deck of cards contains twenty-five cards of five different colors: red, orange, green, blue, and yellow. The same technique is used as with the symbols.

Playing Cards: The next deck of cards is an ordinary set of playing cards. This exercise is very important because the student is again introduced to pictures, colors, and numbers on a white background.

Learning to Read Cards: This deck of cards contains the alphabet and single words. The system for learning to identify these cards is similar to that described for the other decks of cards.

Math Flash Cards: This deck of cards contains math problems. The student learn to see and solve the math problem as soon as the card is flashed by the instructor.

Words and Pictures: This deck of cards contains words and pictures, such as houses, trucks, trains, dogs, cats, and birds. At this point the student is able to see or read a card as fast as it is placed before him or her. There are sixty-five cards in this deck, and some students can identify the entire deck in less than sixty seconds, which is less than one second per card.

Printed Material: At this point the blindfolded student has advanced to the degree that he or she can pick up a book or any printed material and read it as fast as a sighted person.

Learning to expand Visual Field to 360°: Through complete training the student learns to see things above, behind, in front of, or to the side of him or her while blindfolded. This ability is brought about through elementary exercises along with basic ones. There is no standard procedure for teaching, because no two students respond the same way.

Learn to Drive a Car: This ability is enhanced and brought to light through the motion exercises, visual field exercises, and elementary exercises. After the student has learned to see with a 360° visual field and is aware of and can see any motion, he or she is then blindfolded and asked to get behind the wheel of a car. The student is too slowly set the car in motion back and forth until a certain degree of confidence and control is gained. After two weeks the instructor and student select a road in the country that is little used to commence the driving lesson. The student has already acquired the ability to see everything around him or her. All that remains to learn is the distance of motion and stationary objects. After about six weeks of elementary instruction, the student is able to respond to all driving conditions. In fact, unknown to the Washington State Patrol, one student of mine took her driver's test by using her Mind Sight abilities.

Learning to Project One's Mind Great Distances: This exercise actually starts when the student is trained to be placed in another room with the door closed and to identify an object that is in another room. Also the student is placed in a large upright freezer (that has been removed for research) in absolute blackness. The student is blindfolded and then instructed to identify articles placed on the floor outside the box.

As the student's ability to "see" in the distance increases, an instructor monitor every step taken. There can be no error. Someday I hope to be able to project the mind to the far reaches of our galaxy. Sound like wild dreams? It may come about sooner than you think.

Chapter 8

The Training Process

There is a deal of time, love, emotion, effort, and dedication given from the teacher to the student in the training exercises of Mind Sight. The foundation of the entire training exercises is based upon the most noble of all virtues –truth and love. I don't mean the kind of truth that you normally talk about, but truth based on confirmation. I don't mean the kind of love that is based on self and ultimately found to be an illusion, but pure, altruist love that is based on the concept that everything in the universe is connected.

Every step in the process, every action on the part of the trainee must be verified. The techniques are completed by the deep psychological processes that must be understood in order to develop Mind Sight. The trainer must be able to perceive the meaning of the feedback in words and thoughts. Communication between trainer and trainee is physical, verbal, and mental. If the proper communication is not made on all three levels, and if the correct information is not is not passed along the channels of communication between teacher and student, Mind Sight can never be developed. This means that the student must be perceptive, unbiased, completely dedicated to the process, confident that it will work, and ready to evolve by changing old ideas into new ones. The trainee must progress in all levels of mind. Having only one established truth –the truth of love- all relative truth must be verified by their objective function in the real world. That which cannot be verified is treated only as a possibility.

Mind Sight is not just something that can watch other students do, or read about and then simply do unless all the laws, principles, discipline, and faculties are considered. For example, teaching Mind Sight to a sighted person requires certain laws and principles. Teaching persons who are losing their sight or are already blind requires another set of laws and principles. Teaching a person who is blind from birth requires still another. Developing a mainstream of association with permanent and important ideas is required for success with students blind from birth. It is necessary that we make use of idea associations, emotions, or feelings for object impressions. An apple, for instance, is placed before a student and he or she must recall the taste and texture of the fruit; a person enters the room and there is a feeling associated to that person's presence.

During the blind student's training, no idea or impression comes on its own. Sensations and ideas link themselves together to form the real image. For the blind this process is a very difficult one. Without sight, the blind person may put an idea or impression into the mind wholly unconnected to any other idea or sensation, but he or she could never call it again. So we teach the blind person to envision an object or color by trying it to an emotion, idea, feeling, or impression. The rule of thumb is that when there is desire to visualize an object or color frequently, one must associate it with other emotions or ideas that are must likely to come to mind frequently. Logical associations are best.

Training techniques differ from student to student, but basically the result with the blind are the same. After several weeks of specific and regulated exercises there comes an awareness, and then comes an awareness with pure visual sensations completely devoid of significance. The visions are not usually objects existing in and for familiar world, but are colored patches existing in and for themselves, unrelated not only to the external world but also to the student. This kind of awareness last for several weeks, and then a sudden change takes place. The color patches and flashes are no longer sensed merely as colored patches and flashes but become associated with certain objects in external world –especially the color wheel, colored papers, the multicolored ball, hand signals, motion, and papers placed upon the floor. Concentration and attention travels across the visual field of the student's mind, selecting parts of it and perceiving these selected or individual objects as physical objects.

The blind students, Mind Sight is vague and meaningless at first. Eventually it will start to develop into manifestations of definite things belonging to a familiar category situated in an unfamiliar worlds of solid objects until they are recognized and classified by the teacher. Thus perception starts to become clearer; while various details are now perceived for evaluation, other exercises are set in motion. As the new exercises become effective, that which is now apprehended is not merely a set of colored patches or flashes, but a new set of images. For the things seen through the window of the mind are not merely distorted objects, but objects of particular style, color, dimension, or other characteristic. Those characteristics are now perceived, not because the blind have suddenly regained physical sight, but simply because the mind is now in a condition to look for them and to register their significance. The sighted person is also taught to make use of these associations; however, sighted students are fortunate enough to be able to form mental images before they are asked to close their eyes or before they are blindfolded.

Our research shows that 65 percent of people of any of the above classifications can learn Mind Sight if they will only digest what they read in this book. You must have will, faith, and belief to a degree that you never dreamed possible and concentrate to a degree that you think impossible. You must allow your mind to adjust so that you can make it happen.

Chapter 9

To Be a Teacher

One of the most often asked questions of Mind Sight students is, "How can I teach?" I will make and effort to answer this question in this chapter.

Most people can learn Mind Sight but it takes a special person to teach it. Teaching Mind Sight is a concept that defines logic during the teaching and training experience and is so complex that it requires the use of laws, principles, and faculties. Even those who have kept a journal recording the basic exercises or steps still may not qualify to be teachers. The true value of Mind Sight is not always in the storing of factors and principles. You experience them. You experience and study for discipline. You experience and study in order that you, the student, may become the teacher.

In being a student and preparing to be a teacher, you are making yourself fit for the intellectual and motivating encounters of a life in both worlds, so to speak. An educated person, or Mind Sight student, learns to do the things that he or she may not want to do at the time. This type of training helps the student to work into their nerve center. Also by the severe training that the teacher puts to the student, it gives them attention, diversion, mental alertness, and mental control. In other words, the student shall only be what you, the teacher, have prepared them to be. All of the students who have completed Mind Sight say it is all worthwhile because there is nothing in the world so glorious as truth and nothing so fascinating as the pursuit of knowledge and wisdom. The teacher must be mindful that there is in everyone of us a divine curiosity that urges us to inquire for we are put in this world to solve its riddles and mysteries.

We learn because there is something within us, an unquenchable passion, to uncover reality and truth. Mind Sight purifies and exalts the student. It is the bond of time and space, so that one may escape into the infinite and internal. The student must learn that one may unite him or herself with the Creator and establish a oneness with others. It is therefore imperative that a teacher of Mind Sight always listen to, watches, and concentrates on the student during the drills. For every student is an individual and there is something unique about each one. Each student has particular likes or dislikes, desires, problems, and ways of looking at life. But students, as a rule, do not wear their hearts on their sleeves. They do not reveal to every stranger the way in which they differ from others or their hidden abilities. To learn this, the teacher must make an effort to draw the student out so that they will confide in you and allow you to get a glimpse of their interesting characteristics and abilities.

Concentrate and pay attention to all things pertaining to your instruction and to the students acceptance of it. Train yourself to be especially aware of everything that the student reveals in terms of emotions and facial expression and all that is said to you. Advice the student to cultivate good reading and learning habits by repetition. For example, the second reading of a book makes the reader know that book at least three times as well as after the first reading. The importance of repetition in this learning process cannot be overemphasized. It is human nature to become bored or annoyed with what we must repeat over and over, but nevertheless, this must be practiced orally and mentally in order to achieve competence in Mind

Sight skills. No matter how much experience a teacher may have, he or she must always look for additional information that will assist with initial contact with students.

Many a teacher/student relationship is blocked at first because of personality conflicts, or possibly because a teacher lacks psychological knowledge or communication techniques. Unless a teacher is able to successfully establish contact and conduct interviews properly it is a difficult to make progress with the student because of the complexity of the concept. In the first interview, the interest of the student must be awakened. Many a hopeful student will listen to the teacher out of courtesy or curiosity. Such student are often described as disinterested listener, unless the teacher can arouse a genuine interest on the part of the student. Therefore, a teacher must learn that success in any relationship is proportionate to how well the teacher is able to influence the student in following the ideas and the concept. When this is achieved, both teacher and student will be inspired to work together to reach their goal.

A teacher must have personality. The personality is the photograph of oneself that is presented for the inspection of all other personas; it influences others' responses. It is the outward expression of the self – the visible you. The personality can be one's greatest asset if it expresses self-confidence, self-reliance, and sincerity. Personality can also be a liability if it conveys distrust of self, lack of confidence, or insincerity. You can draw people to you or repel them, as you choose. It lies in your hands. You have the same control over your mind that you have over your person. You have the power to acquire those qualities and characteristics that will attract others, assist in convincing and persuading others to agree with you, or enable you to impel others to act as you desire. By power of will a confused thinker can become a careful and clear thinker. Control of the emotions is also possible. Acquiring the determination to develop a personality that will be pleasing and persuading is half the battle. People who lack qualities they need and want are able to develop those qualities through a good Mind Sight teacher.

Staying true to what a person really feels and believes allows one's personality to be influential. Whenever a teacher says the things that are in perfect accord with what he is, then his words have tremendous power to convince and persuade, as well as inspire others to action.

Mind Sight teachers must be constantly aware of the following tools vital for successful teaching.

Study your students: Each person will respond differently to each exercise. Study your student's strengths and weaknesses so you can help them succeed.

Be patient: Always be patient and sensitive with students. Sometimes a student cannot follow your instructions exactly, and it is unpleasant for people to recognize that they cannot perform a desired task.
Remember the power of words: Through words, the teacher stimulates the student to desire Mind Sight, and desire is the most important motivation. Intense desire can brush aside many obstacles.

A teacher must strive to see that the student completes the training. Our reward as teachers is to feel and be a part of the student's success –this is the ultimate test of the teacher's abilities.

EVALUATING STUDENT PROGRESS

1. *Teacher's observation of student:* The teacher observes the student and corrects and evaluates each exercise as it is performed. The teacher also makes a written report of each session.
2. *Video recording:* The teacher makes a videotape from time to time to show the student how others would view his progress. The tapes are kept for student review.
3. *Student journal:* Students are instructed to keep a complete record, or journal, for each session. The following ¿is an example of a student journal.

Dale's Journal 22 March, 1983

Today I could see and was more aware than ever before. I find it very hard to describe exactly what I felt. Light, open free. My block is gone. I believe it was a fear of developing my perception because of what might happen to me when I do. That feat was based on past memories that were finally brought into focus.

That fear is gone now and what is left is an acceptance and assurance of what I am about to experience. I felt like a little girl playing a game that I was winning today. As I went through the exercise and became more and more aware of how much more open I was. I became a delighted child discovering for the first time what play was.

I was very aware of Lloyd at all time and his shadow was consistent. He couldn't lose me at all.

The ball is finally starting to show itself to me in the form of a round glow when I look for it.

The papers were just there at all time; I could ever see the movement of the paper when Lloyd would change it. The colors are there, but sometimes I still see too many at once and have trouble determining which one is in front of me.

We also worked on the eye chart, which is getting bigger. I could pick out each letter as Lloyd asked me to –just by knowing. I'm not quite "seeing" them clearly yet, but the knowing is there along with the visualization. It's like a moving picture in my mind, that I am observing myself.

We worked from the cot again, seeing Lloyds and then the papers. This still was coming in very clear. The door is open, now all I have to do is walk through it.

Dale's Journal 13 April, 1983

I've been away from Mind Sight for two and a half weeks, but things came back clearly for me today. I could see more of the ball and could find it easily. I had a little trouble with the color wheel but I think that was because I had an audience.

Something new started happening today. I had a lot of things in my visual field in the form of overlays. I would see objects all together when they should have been in different places. Something like this:

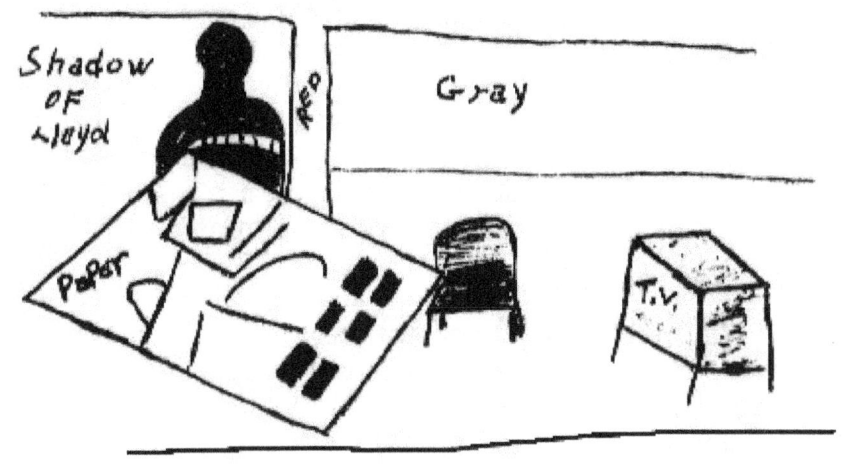

Student's visual field blindfolded

Dale's Journal 14 April, 1983

Today while playing ball with Bill I could see things clearly at times, not just the ball or Bill, but everything around me.

Working with the papers was the same as yesterday, with a lot in my visual field at times. Papers are right there; as soon as I step over one I see the other one, and the image stays rather than fading away.

After several weeks of specific and regulated exercises, Mind Sight is first perceived as a basic awareness. Later, it becomes and awareness with pure visual sensations completely devoid of significance. Objects are not recognized as normal objects existing in the familiar world but as colored patches and flashes existing in and for themselves, unrelated not only to the external world but also to the student. This kind of awareness last for several weeks and then a sudden change takes place. The color patches and flashes are no longer sensed merely as colored images in the external world. These images include colors from the color wheel, colored papers, the ball, hand signals, motion, and papers placed in an orderly fashion on the floor. The student uses concentration and attention to scan the visual field of the mind, selecting certain images and perceiving them as physical objects.

Initially, these perceptions are vague and meaningless, especially to the blind. However, through repetition and concentration, Mind Sight continues to develop until objects begin to be perceived as definite things belonging to a familiar category. For a while, these things will still appear to the student to be situated in an unfamiliar world of solid objects. As the student's perception continues to become clearer and more details are perceived, the teacher introduces new, more advanced exercises to continue to challenge the student's growing perception skills. As the student masters more challenging exercises, his or her mind no longer perceives the outer world as color patches or flashes, but as a set of recognizable images. The objects seen in the mind are not distorted but are identified by a number of distinguishing characteristics such as color, shape, and dimension.

Imagine the excitement of a blind student upon first "seeing" his or her surrounding. Imagine actually being able to read printed material blindfolded. Imagine no guessing, but *knowing*, what lies around you, in the next room, the next building, or the next town.

Chapter 10

Eva's Demonstration

Since I began teaching Mind Sight, I have recruited as many students as I could in order to find out if all people can be taught or just a special person. It turns out that most everyone can be taught. The success rate at first was 15 percent and then it rose to 65 percent and remains at this level today. We gave demonstrations all over the state of Washington to civic clubs, high schools, service clubs, universities, doctors, business men, and churches. In fact, we approached every group that would allow us to demonstrate. Most of the demonstrations during the first two years were given by a student who was the first to succeed in Mind Sight. During this time we experienced things that you would not believe.

One memorable experience was a demonstration at Albuquerque, New Mexico. A newspaper article announced our demonstration as follow:

> A group of scientists will investigate a 'Sightless Vision' demonstration Sunday at the University of New Mexico. The demonstration which is open to the public will be held at the New Mexico Anthropology Hall at 2 p.m. It will be conducted by Lloyd Hopkins of Tacoma, Washington.
>
> Mr. Hopkins has aroused nationwide interest with a program aimed at training people to see without eyes. Mr. Hopkins believes his training

teachings have been refined enough to begin experimental use with blind persons. A panel of scientists and two professional magicians will be on the stage to observe the demonstration. "We have the observers on stage to try and make sure everything is legitimate." said Dr. Henry Monteith. Dr. Monteith is helping coordinate the demonstration. He said a Hopkins trainee is expected to do several things blindfolded, including lighting candles, naming colors, and reading written material. "It is going to be a fascinating program," said Dr. Monteith. "Mr. Hopkins has aroused considerable interest in the scientific community with his work."

Eva Austin, a two year student of Mind Sight, gave the demonstration and mystified the audience in an unforgettable performance. The Albuquerque Times, on Monday, April 29, 1974, printed an article that expressed the emotion and surprise the audience felt. It was a fantastic demonstration.

After this demonstration, a group of scientists in Albuquerque asked if I had ever worked with a person who was blind from birth. I said that I had not but would like to try. Later than summer I was asked to return to New Mexico and was introduced to a nine-year-old girl blind from birth. Arrangements were made for the blind girl to live with us and to attend school near our home. This was to be a pilot program.

After six months of training, the blind girl gave a demonstration al the Sheraton Hotel in Tacoma. Among the invited guests were the Tacoma School

District's teachers for the visually handicapped. Dr. Monteith, who arranged the program with the blind girl, flew in from Albuquerque. The blind girl also gave demonstrations in Seattle, San Francisco, and Albuquerque. Over the years I have worked with many blind students. Many of these students have shown abilities exceeding our research goals.

We have tried to measure these abilities. Two friends of mine who have measuring equipment have made interesting discoveries but found nothing that would prove the existence of Mind Sight to the scientific community. Their measuring devices are inadequate; therefore, they can not scientifically say that Mind Sight exist, even though they witnessed demonstrations many times. One scientist claimed that this was a very humbling fact.

At the moment we are in an amazing learning process. The full abilities of Mind Sight can only be recognized under certain research. This research can be conducted only as we develop the necessary tools and equipment to measure and control it.

Chapter 11

Students Discuss Mind Sight

In his book, *Man's Unconquerable Mind*, Gilbert Highet writes, "People are not born thoughtless or thoughtful. No one can tell how great intellectual minds arise, but when a teacher can detect, they must encourage." At our research clinic in Spanaway, Washington, I conducted extensive research along these lines. I used students with normal senses and, with various methods, was able to develop their sense and intellect beyond what was normal. I gave the students challenges and stimuli, putting problems before them, making things difficult for them in order to create a need to think, and producing things for them to think about so that they would question their thinking at every stage. They were given inventive and original experiments. I asked them to discover what was hidden. I also brought them into contact with other students who had gone through the program. I used challenge, experiment, and association with developed students.

One of the greatest rewards I have found in teaching is to see how students who are stimulated and excited by exploring Mind Sight suddenly begin to change. The students grow in wisdom; They rid themselves of many of their old concepts and beliefs and gain a new understanding of and approach to their abilities, becoming more mature.

MIND SIGHT

> I feel I have scaled the wall of mind
> and as I sit above the beauty of
> what I see,
> I am thrilled with the treasure that
> I find,
> and the wisdom that comes from
> within me.

The above poem was written by Dale Lee, one of my students.

When a student reaches a certain level of awareness, he or she cannot escape the flood of power and knowledge that Mind Sight renders for use.

The following statements have been given before; their importance should be noted again.

> "Man's imagination cannot build a goal too great for him to achieve. Man's controlled thinking can accomplish anything his mind can conceive provided he accepts and believes it."

In this chapter I have asked three students to tell of their experiences with Mind Sight.

DEANNA'S STORY

Recently Lloyd asked me to write something about how I came to be involved with Mind Sight. After eight years of challenges and changes, it's difficult to remember how it really happened.

I once watched "The Helen Keller Story" on television, which described what happened when she was introduced to books. I could understand her thrill and excitement. What wonder to be able to bring the whole world right to you on a piece of paper!

Reading has been my form of experiencing the world around me since I can remember. Nothing "out there" in the world challenged the part of me that books identified.

I've always had a feeling of being guided. It seems that any time I get comfortable, the "school of hard knocks" comes along and drags me away by the ear, as I kick and scream, to new experiences and "trials and tribulations."

Another way that I used to understand my life can be described by this quote from Helen Keller: "The best and most beautiful thing in the world cannot be seen or even touched. They must be felt with the heart." I've always been in awe of life's wonders. No language, art, music, or religion has ever quite been adequate to describe the things my heart knows.

About ten years ago the "school of hard knocks" dumped some books in my lap, which I read. Although I didn't understand the concepts in the books, the idea that they could be taught remained in my mind. Several years later I wrote to a parapsychology research group to inquire if anyone was teaching Huna.

I received a letter putting me in contact with Lloyd. I met with him and began to learn.

Lloyd's training has allowed me to see, understand, and dare more in the last eight years of my life than all the rest of my thirty-seven years. For the first time I can experience life without needing books to translate to me what it is I've experienced. I have found a way to take more control of my life and be in charge of my own direction, although I still do a lot of screaming and kicking. One of the most important things I am learning is how to share with others some of the things I know. By demonstration to the public some of what is possible to learn, I've been giving an opportunity to be involved in teaching others Mind Sight. Also, by never quitting, I am a role model for others. "She learned it, so can I."

A piano teacher who trains a piano soloist with the distinction of an artist like Claude Frank would tell you that, while the teacher had been able to train the majority of his or her students in the fundamentals of piano playing, some students –like Frank- go beyond the fundamentals and become with what they have learned. I think the blind have so strong a desire to see that they will be the people who can be one with their training and best utilize the lessons of Mind Sight in their everyday lives.

A lot of what the mind sees is beyond what can be described, unless there is training to learn to see well enough to describe it. The best way a person can know about Mind Sight is to start the training and learn to see and describe what you see. "Nothing's impossible," says Barbara Streisand. Building on that idea, just think how much there is to see and know.

I learn and grow as a child would. According to child psychologists William Hesson and Katherine Nelson, "Even the youngest infant have a surprisingly organized view of the environment that doesn't depend on language for understanding."

As I read back over these pages, I find I really have no specific events to mark the course of how I came to Mind Sight. My knowing and reading prepared me to be ready for the training that the "school of hard knocks" presented to me when Lloyd accepted me as a student. Job 34:32 say, "That which I see not, teach thou me: if I have done iniquity, I will do no more."

Lloyd's loving guidance and challenges have opened up a whole new world of sight to me. It's a wonderful gift to receive –seeing. I am duplicating the gift and preparing to learn how to teach. I will learn once again as a child with my heart knowing, through reading, and with my newly learned seeing. In this new world of seeing I am a pioneer –a guide to show others the way.

"To dare is our destiny," is the motto of these adventurous students who have learned Mind Sight. I want to find out as much as I can to be a good guide in this world of sights. We've only just begun to explore.

DALE'S STORY

When I met Lloyd Hopkins I had no idea what was in store for me, but what I saw was enough to tell me it would change my life for the better.

In 1979 my family and I moved from California to Washington to follow a dream. I had been studying in the area of psychic phenomena for the past four years and had received a certificate of ministry in the field of metaphysics; yet I felt there had no be another side to all of this –a scientific side. Even though I had strong feelings of the validity of what I had learned I still needed to have proof.

Deanna Calef was my proof in the beginning, but only my own experience gave me the proof I needed. I have always been a positive thinker in that I believe that anything you put your mind to, you can accomplish. You can succeed with time, desire, and training. One of my favorite sayings is, "The measure of a mind's evolution is to accept the unacceptable" by Thea Alexander, from her book, 2150.

Mind Sight to the layman is not believed to be possible, but once you accept the possibility and earnestly work with it you open to yourself a new and exiting world. One of the greatest things I learned from Mind Sight was how important it is, as a student, to put your faith and trust in your teacher; you will find your capacity to learn will be overwhelming. A teacher must be forever patient and understanding of a student in order to gain trust and full attention.

For the student. Mind Sight can be a very rewarding, exciting, and at times, something frustrating experience. It's rewarding in what you learn about yourself. I found a strength in myself that I never realized was there –strength to look at myself as I really am, admit my faults, and revel in the beauty I find in me. You see, it's just as hard to see your qualities as it is to see your faults. As a matter of fact, we have a tendency to dwell on our shortcomings, instead of overcoming them. We must realize our good qualities are what we need to look at and work on. When we do, the faults seems to pass away.

There is nothing more exciting than to experience "seeing" while wearing a blindfold. The most exciting experience I have ever had was when I "saw" a ball rolling across the floor, and I went over and pick it up "seeing" it all the while. This is only the beginning, because once you experience this you feel it should be that way all the time. Unfortunately it's not, and this is the frustration. Just when you think you have "it", you don't. Then your worst enemy –"doubt"- creeps in and you take a few steps back. With the help of your patient teacher, though encouragement, love and positive reinforcement, you continue to make progress until the next big breakthrough and the next "doubting" period.

There will always be a next time because there is no end to the development of Mind Sight. With each new student we learn more, and there will always be someone who will dare to step beyond the restrictions we have placed upon ourselves and bring forth a deeper beauty from within. I sincerely believe that this is what Jesus was trying to teach. After all, didn't he say, "These things I do, you will do also and more"? And we will!

KASSIE'S STORY

I know the reader will identify with almost everything that is said here and understand the theories presented. The only true understanding comes in experiencing a personal knowing that is as individual as are the humans that God made.

As different as our stories may sound, the basic truth remains that man is limited only by his imagination, his faith in himself, and the degree of his desire and belief in his universal purpose.

One must start with a purpose. It can be as simple as to learn, to teach, or to know. I've found desire to be the catalyst. It determines how fast you learn, how hard you work, and how much you want to do it.

In opening your mind, it is hard not to impose new limitations. Truth and faith are words to which attach different meanings. Practicing the meaning is far more difficult. We begin the teaching method by building a foundation on simple truth and expanding that truth; we build a bridge on communication between your conscious and subconscious minds. This will ultimately lead to an understanding of and communication with your superconscious mind. The three must work together in harmony –a mutual bond of trust, faith, and common purpose –to achieve the desired result.

I am always in a hurry, always beginning but seldom finishing. In discipline my mind to take one step at a time, I have found a satisfaction I've never experienced. This simple statement is typical of a point I would like to stress about the individuality of this work. There are many subtle lessons one must realize. They are easy to express in words but often difficult for the individual mind to accept as true. There are many subconscious conflicts; each will be realized when your minds accepts the truth as only it knows it. The truth cannot be hurried or forced upon your conscious mind. It will accept the truth only at its chosen moment. For example, cram for an exam and your mind goes blank when you enter the classroom. You rushed your mind, forcing it to accept the truth which resulted in its own revolution.

I believe everything is possible. I'm now working to find my own truth, believing there is no limit to reality but only levels of awareness. Each level has special responsibilities and I feel compelled to accept the responsibilities in order to fully find the truth of that level of awareness. Often I have found a personal truth in many of the things my teacher has said; I am a reflection of many of his thoughts. Man is the master of the mind, body, and circumstances. Accepting the truth of those words is relatively easy. Our forefathers believed it when they said "All men are created equal." Accepting the responsibility of those words is least difficult when you accept that you are who you are, where you are, and what you are because that is what you chose to be. No one can speak truthfully and excuse their circumstances. You either accept them or change them. You set goals or tasks and either achieve what you desired or are defeated and accept less. It all goes back to finishing what you start.

Excuses are only given by those who fail, and defeat is accepted by those who quit. Therefore man has no limits except those imposed on himself and accepted in his conscious mind. In reality, limits do not exist. I hope you find through reading these pages that you do have a choice of what you are and can find reality in what you want to be.

My being has gone through subtle changes resulting from a series of exercises that seem more like games but are developed especially to heighten one's awareness of things that have always been present. Through exclusion of sight and denial of hearing, my conscious mind has been forced to accept Mind Sight and knowledge that I cannot yet explain. I have found this knowledge to be of such benefit that I look for ways to increase it. In increasing or defining the knowledge I have found my first glimpse of Mind Sight.

Each of my exercises begin with about the same reaction. First there is a struggle within my mind. My conscious mind struggles again new ideas that threaten all that I have been taught in the past. Then when it begins to work, my conscious and subconscious mind begins a series of games that deep concentration and deep realization, with time, can overcome. As the truth of the new idea is presented and proven ever and over again, slowly the two parts of my mind accept this truth. When the conscious mind accepts the truth, the feat is completed, and a second idea can be introduced. If the ideas are submitted too slowly, the mind becomes lazy; and if they are submitted too fast, the mind turns off in revolt.

My exercises in magnetic attraction have progressed from guessing, knowing, feeling, and seeing. The distance and quality of this Mind Sight is under constant improvement. There are times when the attraction is so strong that my hands shake when they are pointed toward my teacher. I feel like the hands of a compass with Mr. Hopkins representing north.

We began work with a series of exercises that were more like games than serious work. In fact, I still have to discipline my mind for concentration. At first reading, one fails to see the importance of these simple exercise, but I caution you to understand that each is important. We often talk about building a stew. We add one thing at a time.

Close your eyes, while standing in the center of a room, hands extended in front of you; your teacher walks around you, stopping from time to time. When he stops you should also stop, with your hands pointing to him. In the beginning, you must force sound from your ears. Standing there with your eyes closed, your conscious mind races to find hints that will tell you where he is. Your hearing is the most developed sense and is the first to be put into use. If you allow hearing, no progress will be made. If you choose not to hear, and to block sound from your conscious, you will soon notice a warmth coming from your teacher's hands. Relax and you will find him.

Exercises are added to expand this new awareness. The student stands with eyes closed and hands in the starting position. The teacher walks at a distance of about eight to twelve feet, pausing while the student points to him and states where he is. Sound must once again be banished from your consciousness. You must never, never peek. It's hard, but soon you will notice that your imagination of where the teacher is gives way to the reality. The warmth is also being expanded to reach out to tell you where he is. The knowing (for I know no other word to explain what it is) tells you where he is.

The third exercise continues the expansion of this knowing. The teacher walks around a large area – fifteen to twenty feet- allowing objects to come between himself and you. Reinforcing the loss of sight and sound forces the conscious mind to use its new awareness to find the teacher. This results in expansion of the depth of awareness and the ability to be exclusive, picking out the teacher instead of other objects. In the beginning, imagination may be all that you have, but soon this will give way to reality.

These first three exercises are basic. They form the foundation for anything to come in the future. They are performed every time the teacher and student meet. During the months, subtle changes in response to these exercises will act as a barometer for the teacher. As these changes in awareness show themselves, additional exercises will be added to the learning period.

I should now tell you about the other exercises I have participated in, and tell you about my feelings. I will review these exercises, telling you how my response to them has changed.

Colors are introduced by means of live color. We use a color wheel with the four basic colors –red, green, yellow, and blue. The color wheel moves in any direction, which makes it impossible to count rotations in order to know the color. At first you close your eyes, looking directly at the color wheel, with the lights in the room turned off. You are introduced to the colors and asked to the wheel the color bath your whole being. Soon you will notice that the color is penetrating your eyelids. To compensate for this the student is asked to turn his or her head so as not the face the light. You proceed by turning your back to the lights and finally using a blindfold.

At first I guessed the colors, and I was surprised at what happened. There I would sit, listening to the whir of the motor turning the wheel, and imagining the colors passing in front of me. When the wheel would stop, I would open my mouth to say a color and something else would come out. Surprisingly that "something-else color" would be right. I do not know how my subconscious knew the colors and told my conscious. Sometimes I would know the next color before the wheel began to run. I learned to trust this knowing and I rely on it even now in this exercise and others. Also, the colors had a feel or an emotional association. Blue was sad, yellow was happy, red was hot, and green was cool. One day, the colors came right through the blindfold and did bath my whole being. I didn't see the colors on the wheel, but the inside of my mask would glow with the color as they changed on the wheel. Today, it is a combination of seeing and knowing, or sometimes only one or the other.

We began to add to our add exercises. I would stand in a corner, and my teacher would walk to a position and stop: I would say, where he was. He then placed three papers between us. I would walk from my position to his with my eyes closed trying to point to the papers as I passed them. There were a couple of physical obstacles to overcome. Balance is changed, and confidence in your ability to walk is altered. Right now, close your eyes and walk from where you are sitting to the door and back. See what I mean? You really want to peek, but don't! Your desire to find Mind Sight will help you to your breakthrough. I also found it difficult to walk to where I was pointing. Papers were added after confidence had been gained. At first it's guessing, and the teacher responds by correcting errors. Through practice you will find that your guessing becomes more of a knowing.

There are many papers exercises, all of which are introduced about the same time. I must stress that you should not peek and that you should relax. I have found that if I relax and wait for Mind Sight to come, I have an impulse to look or listen. Sometimes the impulse is so strong that it is almost a panic. If you resist the panic, Mind Sight will come as this lostness subsides. If it doesn't come right away, I find a paper and look at it closely –its shape, whether it is soiled, whether it has corners. I close my eyes slowly, concentrating on it and saying yes, yes, yes, while I reach down and touch it. My imagination of that paper is changed into reality as I touch the paper which is the proof of that reality. Accepting one truth, I go to the next. If it's not there, immediately I fight peeking and begin repeating yes until I touch it. As I touch it, I again reinforce the truth, changing imagination into reality. It comes easier with each paper.

I've found the papers to be the vehicle of my greatest learning and cause for my deepest despair. As we began my search for a mental vision of papers, I looked for anything I could use as a clue to their location. The whiteness I looked for would move or float up out of sight as I reached down to verify the truth. At times it would appear and disappear much like a strobe light. And at times it would be entirely wrong. The way I experienced the papers, the way I saw them from day to day, in the beginning, was not always the same. What my subconscious mind saw was denied by my conscious mind as pure fantasy, and it fought for its exclusive right of sight.

I must tell you about the games my mind has played with me. I can now feel the conflict going on within my consciousness. I feel you must work in harmony with the conscious and subconscious doing their own particular jobs, neither leading nor following. Now I'm aware of the conflict before it manifests itself as a game.

The true Mind Sight I've experienced seems to drift in form somewhere above my head. Everything appears phosphorescent. At first it's difficult to judge heights, because everything is floating and somewhat out of perspective. The sight does not come from the eye sockets as we are used to, but from another point. This point of vision I am not yet able to control but accept gladly, however it wants to come. I will learn to see it with practice.

I sometimes find my "sight" floating out of the picture. It's easer to keep sight when the picture changes as in identifying cards, colors, or objects, or in walking about. But, then it goes as it came and all is black as though I walked into a closet and someone slammed the door closed behind me. This experience happens so quickly it almost takes your breath away. Just wait and it will come back. I don't know if every student's experiences are the same. These are mine.

I feel that Mind Sight is something so subtle that it is always present with all people but overlooked. Our minds have been so filled with limits, that much work must now be undertaken to bring back those abilities that we were given so long ago.

Chapter 12

Practical Applications Of Mind Sight

One does not need to be a Christian to be a student of Mind Sight, but one must have the desire and will to seek new knowledge, the belief and faith to accept it, and the will to use one's faculties to the limit. It is a shame that a few religious students who failed in the program have said, in effect, that if God had wanted them to learn Mind Sight he would have made it possible. The fact is that the student blamed his or her laziness and weakness on God. It seems we are always looking for a scapegoat when the going gets tough. Unfortunately, not everyone can achieve Mind sight, for various reasons; but God is not one of these reasons. The reasons can be illness, lack of faith and belief in oneself, lack of vital force, the inability to comprehend, and other pressing problems of a personal nature –but never God.

Mind Sight, in a way, is similar to the way science was described by one of the hosts of the television program, "Nova".

> "Science may not be perfect; it is only a tool which could be misused, but as I look around I find it is the best tool we have. With this tool we are self-correcting and ever-changing. The important thing is that with this tool we can vanquish the impossible."

Mind Sight is not trying to introduce a new religion but to awaken the reader to what we have and to separate legend and truth –and through this to build upon truth.

I firmly believe that many of my students, and myself, are at the doorway of a room filled with life's most precious treasure –the ability to see even for those without eyes and the ability to see and experience the hidden possibilities of the mind. But the doorway is just partially open. Only a few have stepped through and even they, although demonstrating what appears to others as superhuman powers, have only begun to touch their potential.

In order to research all the abilities that Mind Sight can offer, we need many volunteers –doctors, scientists, teachers, students, including students of religion. And, of course, we need a place to work and money for equipment for monitoring our progress. But most important we need many volunteers to learn to teach and be teachers of the concept.

Dr. Henry Monteith, a scientist with Scientific Laboratories in New Mexico, examined demonstrations that he conducted and his own experiences and noted the practical application of Mind Sight.

1. "Developing the ability in the blind to "see" with even greater accuracy than those with normal vision.

2. Contributing greatly to a further understanding of man –his purpose, nature, and science.

3. Improving the creative thinking of all people who make use this method.

4.   A value beyond measure in developing the latent potential of children. Indeed, it can be applied with children more easily than it can with adults.

5.   There is no limit as to what can be accomplished in education. Special notice should be given to the following issues.

>   A.   The child of Mind Sigh, what will he become?
>
>   B.   A new light in modern science.
>
>   C.   Ultimate uses of Mind Sight.
>
>   D.   Mind Sight in love, courtship, and marriage.
>
>   E.   Creative and fundamental brain centers.
>
>   F.   Application of Mind Sight to social questions.
>
>   G.   Mind sight and its relation to true religion.
>
>   H.   Mind Sight and its application to higher education.
>
>   I.   The final discoveries in Mind Sight: Where will it take man?"

"The one thing that we discovered in Mind Sight is that we have only scratched the surface of a remarkable phenomena of mind. Not one of us knows what Mind Sight contains. Not one of us knows what Mind Sight can or will do."

All we do know is that it is an accepted concept. It demonstrate with physical proof that it can witness all the laws, principles, and faculties of perception.

"The ancient prayer of the Kahuna from the temple tower was 'Let that which is unknown become known.'"

It is common knowledge that every human mind is filled with unused abilities and power. Yet very few of us attempt to learn to use this great power.

At the outset of my discovery of Mind Sight, it was heartbreaking going through all the trial and error. Now that I have learned to use all the laws, principles, faculties, disciplines, vital force, and psycho-physical skills, it looks so simple. Yet the question still remains. What will it take to find man's true potential? When the body is sick, it cries out to be healed. Does the mind cry out to be whole?

There are two areas of my research that may lead to greater knowledge and expand Mind sight research to the next step or level. The first is to project Mind Sight beyond the psycho-physical level to a pure mental level. Second, we must learn to use the mind as a time machine so that we can move ahead to a future goal and lock in on that goal, mentally and physically as we do in Mind Sight –not subconsciously, but concisely until the mission is accomplished. The choice to stay or return is ours.

The same thing applies to a point in history. Lock in, explore, and experience all the mind and body can offer. We must explore, in truth, our origin. What are the true facts of the past? Can we see beyond the far reaches of our galaxy?

These experiments in accuracy and truth can only be accomplished for those who have accomplished Mind Sight on our teaching level; for only they have learned to differentiate between imagination and reality. I have experimented in these areas for the past ten years to record their practicability. Now I am certain it can be done.

I know this may sound far-fetched, but I heard on a "Nova" program that "we are creatures of curiosity seeking ourselves. We have no idea of our true place in the universe. There are so many things to explore, that the human mind shall never be lacking for fresh knowledge."

The amazing value of Mind Sight is that, once learned, it can be used as a step in any direction for research. It is like standing in the center of a huge retunda onto which a thousand doors open. The question is, which door will you open next?

There is no way of knowing where the next great discovery will come from, since most discoveries began as a dream of impossibility. The new discoveries in science demonstrate that man is a progressive being, and his progression in the direction of self-knowledge, which is the essence of all knowledge, has been accelerated to a rapid pace. The intellect of man is taking a wide view of the whole of man.

Yet the world of the mind seems to be in a state of change and commotion. Although trying to hide from the truth, we learn some of its secrets by accepting each mental exercise as one of the manifestations of its functional activity. This points to the conclusion that a definite order must be observed. In other words, the order of steps or exercises had to be followed or there is no progress.

Chapter 13

Advanced Research

The whole field of Holistic medicine is being brought into a new focus as a legitimate area of science for professional study. Knowledgeable people are finding so many times in many areas, questions that have long been unexplained by traditional science are now being explored in hopes of finding the answers.

Our research has produced results that no other research in the country, or perhaps the world, to our knowledge has produced. We have had doctors and scientists from the world over visiting our center and viewing our results.

Through continued research I hope to contribute my part to help man-kind to find himself to be whole. To be a whole person will require more open-mindedness and understanding than ever before. Young students particularly should have an immediate and imperative need to learn new abilities to help all who wish to improve their skills and abilities.

I have designed a program not only to aid students in bringing about his present possibilities and abilities, but also to help him or her to continue to improve upon the concept at hand. I will continue to stimulate the student to create greater responses by presenting more challenging material. Prompting him or her by open-minded discussions, and directing them by pointing out their success in Mind Sight.

In selecting certain goals for my continued research, my first consideration is to start with a hypothesis in certain areas that are still baffeling to science, by using information and understanding now available to me from Mind Sight. This information will enable myself and the student to comprehend more of the phenomenon in the work ahead.

Excluding Mind Sight, but, by using information in its findings, I have sought out several practical areas. Areas I believe would be adaptable to the present needs of science, interested students, and myself. The student, while working in Mind sight, would choose the order according to his or her own abilities and skills.

I realize there are so many areas of equal importance but I feel I should stick to the areas my research has couched on before. The order of nature from the beginning of the time down to the present day has been that knowledge or change does not come on a silver platter, but be fought for inch by inch against bigotry, abuse, and ignorance. Yet there is one excellent feature about Mind Sight in contrast with other systems of mental philosophy. It not only helps us to expedite the expressions we hold by nature and varied abilities we posses, but it also teaches direct methods of rectifying mental blocks by demonstrating how man can do his part in promoting the ultimate perfection in his make-up. This is the grand value of Mind Sight. It will perhaps find the best of all men, and reveal how it may be developed to even greater heights.

Our demonstrations and the work printed here are an encouragement for all who are seeking to make the best use of their lives and mental powers.

Chapter 14

Mind Power Discovery

Before the discovery of Mind Sight, I tried all the available knowledge around. It didn't aid in the discovery of Mind Sight, but it was a lot of fun. I learned Mind Sight Control through my investigations in hypnosis, psychometric analysis, clairvoyance, psychokinesis, and levitation, as well as mental telepathy and astrol projection. In fact, I did so well in most of these areas that I have in my files many newspapers articles and letters from universities where I demonstrate mind power. I don't demonstrate abilities when compared with Mind Sight.

But to give the reader an idea of what I received from Mind Power, I will explain some of the demonstrations. One day I was invited to give a demonstration of Mind Power at a community college. In addition to using the basic things like hypnosis, I decided to use a new approach that I had been working on –an association by awareness and magnetic association. This is a means of developing sensation between teacher and student or any two people. In a short time the magnetic attraction got so strong that the subject could feel and respond to the magnetic pull up to forty feet. This can be developed to many times that distance now. In fact, I had the audience completely surround me, yet my subject could pick me out the crowd blindfolded. This is one exercise I use in Mind Sight today.

At another demonstration I was invited by Dr. John Wilmarth of O.V.T. to speak of mind projection of Mind Sight and a teacher asked me if was possible to project a person's mind to a certain place. "Well, no," I said. "I have not accomplished that yet to a demonstration level. I and to a point where I can project a mind, but I must follow through to validate this particular situation."

The teacher agreed to be the subject. After talking with her for a few seconds I said, "Now, where are you?" She said she was looking around. "All right. I am going to send Dr. Wilmarth from the building and I want you to follow him. Wherever he goes I want you to tell me his every move." Dr. Wilmarth left the building and went over to the main office and then to the flag pole and stood close to the flag pole. Dr. Wilmarth came back and verified what had happened. She had told the audience, what he was doing. It was through this demonstration and this teacher's effort that I was able to confirm my new avenue of projecting the mind on another person. This was another secret and the first real opportunity I had to demonstrate this ability.

Dr. Wilmarth called me the next day and said there were a couple of people who wanted to talk with me. One of the girls was the teacher that I used in the demonstration of mind projection. The other was a student. They said that they would like to learn more about what I was doing. I told them to "join the crowd."

I started working with this teacher. In Mind Sight I found that I could not only teach, but that she could learn in a very short time what I had covered. It kept me busy progressing all the time, because I would never try to put a student through something that I didn't go through myself. I had to know if there were any side effects.

When acting as a subject and teacher at the same time I would use a tape recorder and often times my wife would help me. The first time I saw the paper I knew that I had breakthrough. It only took me about three months to see the paper, but it took six months to figure out how I had seen it or what steps created the breakthrough. There are forty-two steps in Mind Sight, but I did not know the number of steps at that time. I did know that they had to follow in sequence. One had to follow the other or it would not work. I found this out later.

One day a doctor questioned me about a demonstration I gave regarding mind control.

Q. What did you tell them about losing weight?

A. That this more or less is mind control, or a physical control by the mind. We are capable of giving ourselves commands that can be carried out if we really believe and have the will to carry out the command that we give ourselves. The mind will give you nothing on a silver platter. We must earn it and this is what I am trying to teach –that all things are possible by belief, faith, will, and simple suggestions. To lose weight I pretty much give the same instructions I gave you. First, stand in front of a mirror nude. Look at yourself. Ask this question. Is this the person you really want to be? Get a photograph of yourself at an earlier time when you were slim and trim. Look at these two pictures. Which one would you prefer? Which one do you really want to be? If your desire and the other factors I mentioned above are strong enough, you will make the transition.

Q. What do you mean by that?

A. You lose weight. I had a class of about 20 students, and at the time I weighted 216 pounds. To demonstrate weight mind control, I agreed to lose one pound per day for thirty days. In fact, at the end of thirty days I had lost thirty-six pounds.

Q. Did you quit eating?

A. No. I ate regularly, three meals a day, sometimes four, and I still eat that many.

Q. Was physical exercise involved?

A. I would get in front of a mirror and strip down to my underclothes. I would use certain calisthenics to tone up the body, allowing the mind to do all the physical work. I would just go through the motion, allowing the mind to concentrate on each movement so hard that I could actually feel the muscles pull from the simple exercise

Q. Well, do you do knee bends over the head?

A. I do hands on hips, hands over the head, extending the hands out, the hands in front, then I move my arms back and forth, and often times I do knee bends. I walk about two or three times per day. This is for leg and back tone. This was the doctor's recommendation after back surgery.

Q. How long a time do you spend in front of a mirror to lose weight?

A. The weight? I don't do that anymore. I have been at 172 lbs. For the past eight years.

Q. But how much time did you spend in front of a mirror each day to lose weight?

A. Perhaps a half hour, repeating the suggestions I wanted to take hold. "Reduce the flab. Take it off. I don't need it." I kept telling my mind that this was something that I did not need, I did not want. It was unhealthy and it looked ridiculous. I made the affirmations with such strength , belief, will, and faith that it took hold.

Q. How much time did you spend on the exercise?

A. I spent about seven minutes a day in exercises.
Q. Do you tense the muscles any?

A. I do. I tense the muscles and then I allow the mind to take over or take hold to bring the pressure, to bring the pull and strain. I don't say I am lazy, but this is more rewarding to me than weight lifting.

Chapter 15

Kirlian Photography

In 1973 I read an article in a magazine regarding research being carried out by Dr. Henry Monteith, in the area of Kirlian photography. It illustrated a camera that was developed by Henry to take Kirlian pictures. I was so interested in this new approach that I went to the University of New Mexico where Henry was researching this concept. Over lunch we discussed each other's research.

I learned from Henry that Kirlian photography was developed in Russia by two Russian scientists – husband and wife team- Samyon and Valentina Kirlian, around 1939. Henry was introduced to this technique in 1970 at a symposium he attended in Czechoslovakia. Henry, after hearing of my research was interested in how my students would photograph during Mind Sight training.

Henry passed on to me the results of his study to date. He also sold to me a new machine designed to take Kirlian photographs for research work. I have used this technique in an experimental way since 1974, and have had a number of visits with several researchers to expand my knowledge of this technique

I have been able to predict success and failure in Mind Sight students based on my evaluation of their Kirlian photographs. I have also worked with two medical doctors in comparing a student's photographs with their known illness. While no statistical correlation studies were made, the evidence suggests that if a standardized technique were developed on the part of medical researchers using standardized equipment, film, and time, the validity of the technique could be determined. This lack of standardization has hindered any studies confirming the work of other researchers. However, my success in predicting successful achievement in Mind sight has given me confidence in the technique as I used it.

While it would probably take a college course to thoroughly explain Kirlian Photography, the same could be said of a new student to psychology. But in order to make the reader acquainted with the technique as practiced here, the following is a summary of our use of Kirlian photography.

I was discovered by the Kirlians that an electric charge of high voltage and low amperage applied to a finger would cause a discharge of electrical energy around the finger that could be photographed in different colors. This cold be accomplished in a dark surrounding by touching a piece of undeveloped photographic film with the electrically charged finger. Photos vary with the person according to his or her state of health, personality, state of tension, and feelings or emotions at the time the photo is taken. Other factors also enter into the way the photo energy is transferred to the negative. The study made of the thousands of pictures I have taken over the last fourteen years, has helped me to develop a personal method of evaluating these photographs, as a means of identifying the student to me and to himself. It is not only a lot of fun for the student, but a challenge in researching new discoveries for Kirlian users.

Chapter 16

Students to Remember

Why is Mind Sight to unique? The main reason is that, unlike others who claim to have abilities from birth, or those who say they developed the ability in their lifetime, we are able to teach individuals this ability. This fact makes this work significant for all of those who have the undeveloped potential to use Mind Sight.

Today, as I reflect over the past fifteen years, I recall the fantastic student that I have worked with. They were from all walks of life. The students were taught to do the basic exercises. Beyond these, they were taught more advanced skills, such as driving a car while blindfolded, reading printed material, seeing in complete detail all objects within several miles, reading letters in an unopened envelope while blindfolded, describing pictures in full detail at a twenty feet distance, and much, much more.

Yet, among all the students who demonstrated, there were a few who were outstanding. One such student – in fact my first student to see without eyes- was a teacher ay Olympia Technical Institute in Olympia, Washington. Her name was Eva . She was an exceptional beautiful person. Eva gave over thirty demonstrations to civic clubs, professional clubs, schools, scientific communities, and universities. Eva was gracious, beautiful, and was an inspiration to other students by her demonstration in grace and perfection. We had no founding, and she bought gowns for the demonstration with her own money.

Eva, a teacher in Computer Technology is the first student I taught to see without eyes.

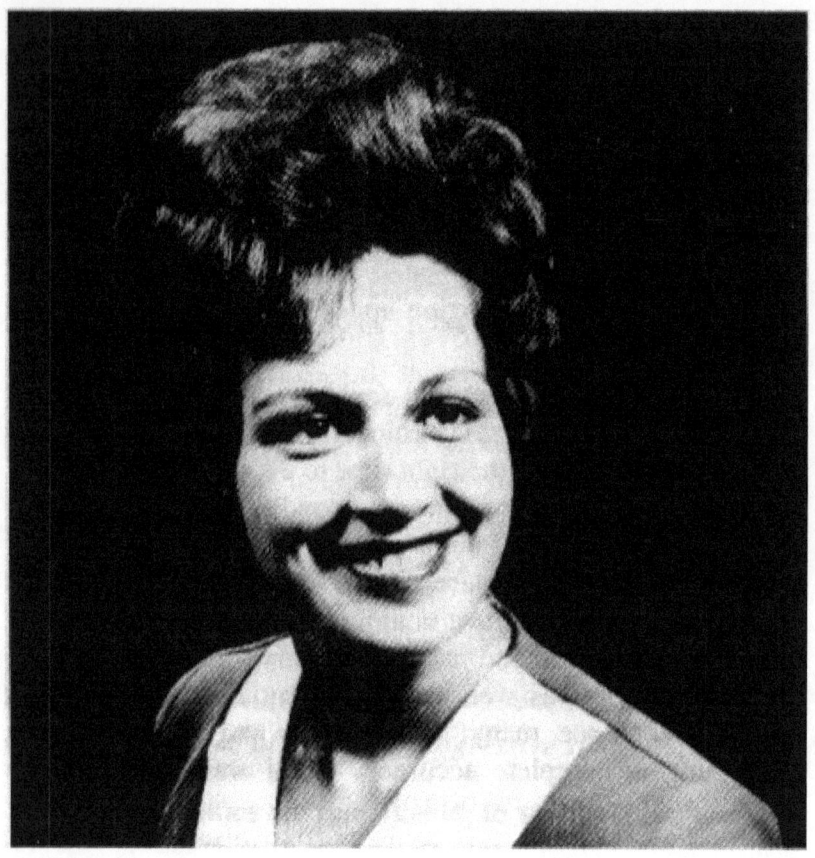

While blindfolded, Eva could see things over her head, such as balloons, read printed material in unopened envelopes, and see at great distance. She gave a superb demonstration at the University of New Mexico for a panel of scientists. Without this student's demonstration, there would be no Mind Sight today. I shall always be indebted to this girl.

KASSIE: She also was a student who took great pride in her work and gave many demonstrations in perfection. She was a very pretty girl and had a love for knowledge and the unknown. Kassie gave a television demonstration in Tacoma, Washington for schools and civic clubs and learned to drive a car blindfolded. Kassie also demonstrated for scientists and was inspiration for new students.

CLARA: Clara could always be dependent upon for any kind of a demonstration. She assisted me in working with two blind students. Clara was attractive, very popular with the students, and loved to demonstrate. She gave several demonstrations to the psychology class at Pacific Lutheran University for Dr. Jessie Nolph. She demonstrated for high schools and civic clubs and had three television appearances for major Seattle stations.

She had basic abilities. She could read while blindfolded, drive a car blindfolded, play chicken (that is, drive toward an object, then veer off at the right time to avoid a crash), and she could demonstrate under abnormal conditions. In one demonstration, she read fro a book while in a leather hood over her head, and when cards were put on a distant table, she read every card right. She gave demonstrations for instructors of the visually handicapped and for scientists. She developed her ability to see many, miles away and could describe everything in complete accuracy. Clara was almost totally blind.

MARY: She was an excellent demonstrator, although she was not with us for very long. Her husband who was in the Army, was transferred to another country.

DEANNA AHD HER DAUGHTER CRISTI: They started working with me several years ago. They gave several

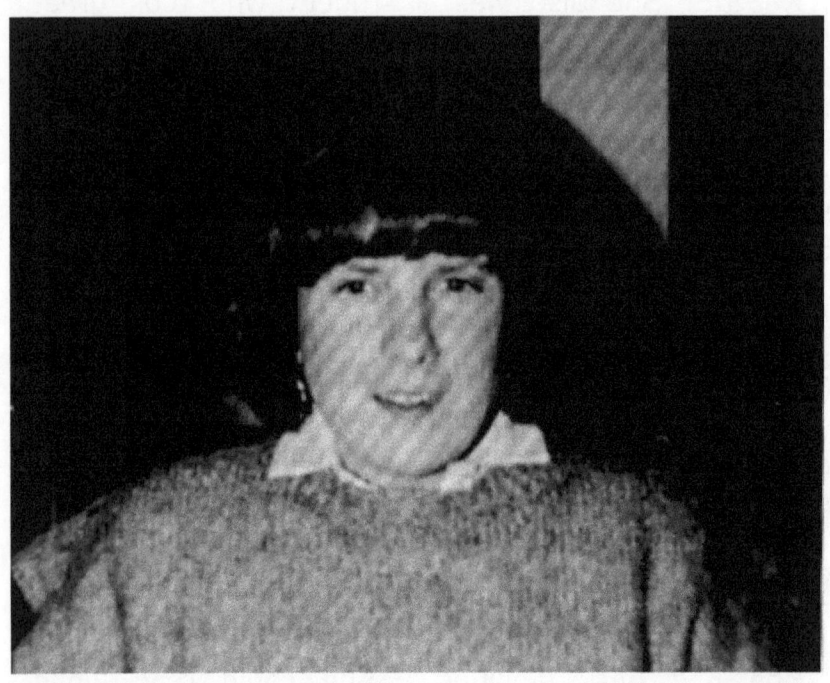

demonstrations for civic groups, schools, and television. Cristi was only nine when she started working and dropped out to continue school.

Deanna, one of our most progressive students.

Deanna is a nurse and supervisor at Western State Hospital. She has given many demonstrations to hospitals, civic groups, and medicals, and gave two demonstrations for the American Holistic Medical Association –the Northwest Chapter. She has also demonstrated for doctors from foreign countries, television, schools, universities, religious groups, the King County Blind Association, and the Pierce County Blind Association (of which she is an honorary member).

Deanna's abilities are remarkable, to say the least. She will soon demonstrate in an area never seen in public before.

DALE: Dale was our office secretary, and donated almost all of her time. Dale was a student in Mind Sight for over a year and a half. She is also a minister. Dale is a very pretty girl and learned fast. She was helped put on demonstrations, assisted in making a video, did liaison work, and, all in all, was her our girl Friday. At the death of her mother, she left for California to be with her father. We love her very much and wish her well. Hopefully, she will return to continue her training. Her training would be an asset to her profession. God be with you, Dale, wherever you go.

BILL: Bill is a retired air force lieutenant colonel and has a PhD in human behavior. Bill took the training with great success. He was a professor in psychology and other disciplines. He was very active in most of the activities concerning the welfare of Mind Sight. He arranged demonstrations and was the overseer of office procedures.

We have worked with many blind students in a pilot program funded by my personal funds. Some are blind as a result of accidents, illness, or diabetes; others are blind from birth, Several newspapers articles have been written regarding their progress and success. It is their response to Mind Sight that created the need to write this book –to show that Mind Sight may be the key to opening their minds to a sight once known or to a sight never known.

My pilot program came to a halt because of a lack of founds. To continue this pilot program we need help in founding. I realize there is a large cost in both time and money, but it's worth it.

Read some of the accomplishments that these proud people have achieved.

A NINE-YEAR-OLD-GIRL: Blind from birth, in six months time, she was able to identify colors on the color wheel. She could give proper orientation and color paper placed upon the floor. She gave many demonstrations. Her story is covered in other chapter.

ANNIE: A seventy-three year-old lady, legally blind, she developed the ability to identify colors from the color wheel, colors of papers, cards, objects, symbols, and read from an eye chart. She gave two demonstrations. One of these was for KingTV in Seattle, Washington and the other for a professional from the Veterans Administration Hospital in Steilacoom, Washington –both with a blindfold on.

ROCKY: He was completely blinded as a result of a car accident. Rocky is one of our very special students. I am sure his story is being written by his doctor through his medical exams.

We had a lady blind from birth that offers a story of dedication likened to Helen Keller's experience. There are no words that can truly describe this lady. For several years she worked with Deanna and me. The hardships she endures to keep her commitment are remarkable. For example, she lives about a mile and a quarter from the bus line in Seattle and walks every Monday (rain or shine) to the bus stop, travels to downtown Seattle and transfers to a bus to Federal Way. We pick her up in Federal Way and take her to the Federal Way library to practice. Sometimes she misses her bus connection and waits, sometimes over an hour, for another bus. She does all this no matter if it rains, sleets, snows, or is sunny.

This lady is married to a most wonderful and understanding person. Although she is not consistent yet, she has given many demonstrations. She also demonstrated for our documentary commercial video tape.

We have been working with several doctors in different disciplines and are near breakthrough level. There are many more helpful students –too many to mention at this writing.

It is my hope that science will not overlook this new challenge and will provide the necessary funds and monitoring equipment to continue this special human research.

Chapter 17

Conclusion

Today, Mind Sight is accepted as a serious study more than it was when I developed the concept eighteen years ago. Each day our society advances in knowledge. I often consider how lucky we are to live during this period in time when we are delving into the great mysteries of the past and are experimenting with present perceptions for future reality.

The mechanism by which Mind Sight is learned is not hypnosis or any of the occult sciences. It is a structured teaching process. Through our research, we have come to believe that this learning process light the way to opening many doors of mind. The concept certainly merits further serious exploration

It is true that some of my research has been attributed to areas of parapsychology. However, as a serious researcher, I was interested only in the natural order of things. We believe the super, or above the normal, is only defined by limited experience.

I, like others, am probing for answers to universal questions. What is our true role and power in life? Where did we come from? Why are we here? Where are we going?

I have learned that we all have the abilities to obtain greater understanding, knowledge, and wisdom; but we often do not know enough to use our power or abilities. The average person is almost totally unaware of his mental powers that remain undiscovered for a simple reason –fear.

I have been studying and experimenting in this area for approximately eighteen years, and I will be the first to admit I have barely opened the door to magnificent possibilities. In fact, science tells me that I have stumbled upon the fringes of a new truth that could have value beyond measure in science, education, medicine, advances for handicapped, and for the future development of the human mind.

Mind Sight today is a solid concept because it demonstrate with physical proof what we are all capable of. It stands as a witness and challenge to belief, faith, and faculties of perception.

Eyeless sight is not only possible, it can be demonstrated repeatedly with 100 percent accuracy. Think what Mind Sight can mean to us, to our children, and especially to those who are visually handicapped. A whole new world is available to these people, and it's up to all of us to open the doors wide.

I am not psychic, nor were any of the people who worked with me. Our hope is that after you read this book, you can share the thrill and hope of this new world in your own experiences. I read somewhere, "The greatest friend to truth is time, her greatest enemy is prejudice, and her constant companion is humility."

Bibliography

Love and Wisdom, *Richard Hubler*
Crown Publishers, Inc., New York, NY
Copyright 1968

Deanna's Story, *Deanna*

Secret Science Behind Miracles, *Max Freedom Long*
DeVorsa & Co. Publishers, Los Angeles CA 90041
Copyright 1948- 1949

Man's Unconquerable Mind, *Gilbert Highet*
Columbia University Press, New York, NY
Copyright 1954

Origin of Species, *Charles Darwin*
New American Library Reprint 1953

Practical Applications, *Dr. Henry Monteith*

Kassie's Story, Given for this publication

The Kahuna, *by L.R. McBride*
The Petroglyph Press, Hilo, Hawaii

Dale's Journal, *by Dale*

Dale's Story, *by Dale*

Where to Order this Book

(1) You can order online from Amazon.com at:

http://www.amazon.com

Search for this book by title or by the ISBN number:

ISBN-13: 978-1-884979-01-9
ISBN-10: 1-884979-01-7

(2) For wholesale or bookstore orders, go to Ingram Book Group

http://www.ingrampublisherservices.com/retailer/default.asp

One Ingram Blvd.
P.O. Box 3006
LaVergne, TN 37086-1986

(866) 400-5351

Retailer@ingrampublisherservices.com

For all other inquiries, contact the publisher by logging onto the website and using the contact form.

Published by:Clear Springs Press, LLC
Yelm, WA   U.S.A.
http://www.clspress.com/contact.html

www.ingramcontent.com/pod-product-compliance
Lightning Source LLC
Chambersburg PA
CBHW031156160426
43193CB00008B/397